Alton's Antibiotics and Infectious Disease

ALTON

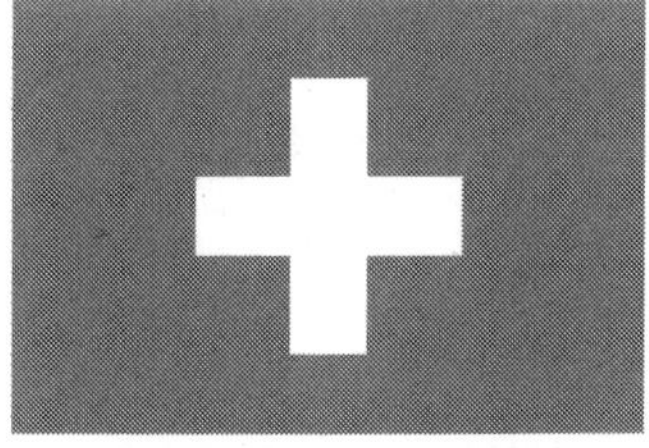

FIRST AID

AN ALTON FIRST AID GUIDE

Alton's Antibiotics and Infectious Disease

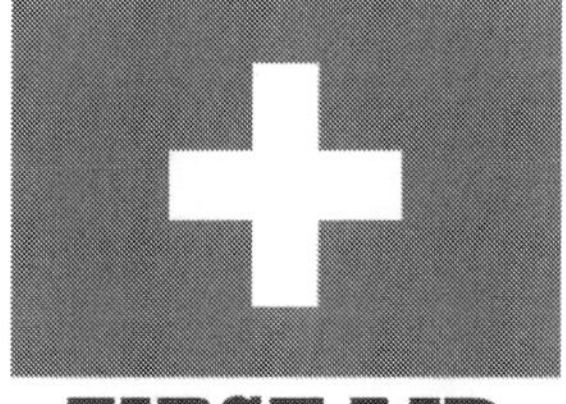

THE LAYMAN'S GUIDE TO AVAILABLE ANTIBACTERIALS IN AUSTERE SETTINGS

JOSEPH ALTON MD
AMY ALTON ARNP

DISCLAIMER

All information in this book is meant for educational and entertainment purposes only and does not constitute medical advice nor the practice of medicine. No provider-patient relationship, explicit or implied, exists between the publisher, authors, and readers. This book does not substitute for such a relationship with a qualified provider.

As many of the strategies discussed in this volume would be less effective than proven present-day medications and technology, the authors and publisher strongly urge their readers to seek modern and standard medical care with certified practitioners whenever and wherever it is available.

The reader should never delay seeking medical advice or disregard medical advice because of information in this book. Neither should the reader begin, adjust nor discontinue any medical treatment because of information in this book or any resources cited by this book.

Although the authors have researched all sources to ensure accuracy and completeness, they assume no responsibility for errors, omissions, or other inconsistencies therein. Neither do the authors or publisher assume liability for any harm caused by the use or misuse of any methods, products, instructions or information in this book or any resources cited by this book.

Photographic images by Amy Alton, Shutterstock

Printed in the United States of America

ISBN-13: 978-0-578-41452-2

DEDICATION

This book is dedicated to the people who keep others healthy in austere settings without access to the miracle of modern medicine. We hope this book serves to empower these brave individuals in their efforts to save lives that would otherwise be lost.

JOSEPH ALTON MD, FACS, FACOG

AMY ALTON ARNP, CNM

"Do what you can, with what you have, where you are..."

—THEODORE ROOSEVELT

ABOUT THE AUTHORS

Joseph Alton MD, FACOG, FACS practiced as a board-certified Obstetrician and Pelvic Surgeon for close to 25 years before retiring to devote his efforts to preparing families medically for disaster scenarios. A Life Fellow of the American College of Obstetrics and Gynecology and retired Fellow of the American College of Surgeons, he is a contributor to many well-known preparedness, survival, and homesteading magazines. He also serves as a speaker at preparedness conferences throughout the country on the subject of medical readiness. A member of MENSA, Dr. Alton collects medical books from the 19th century to gain insight on off-grid medical strategies.

Amy Alton ARNP, CNM is an Advanced Registered Nurse Practitioner and a Certified Nurse-Midwife. She has had years of experience working in large teaching institutions as well as smaller, family-oriented hospitals. She is the designer of a popular line of quality first-aid and trauma kits available at store.doomandbloom.net. Amy is dedicated to providing medical education and the highest level of customer service and satisfaction.

Dr. and Ms. Alton are both certified Advanced Wilderness Expedition Providers (AWEP) and the founders of an award-winning survival medicine website at doomandbloom.net. They are also the co-authors of the 1st place winner of the Book Excellence Award in medicine "The Survival Medicine Handbook: The Essential Guide for When Medical Help is Not on the Way." As "Dr. Bones and Nurse Amy," they host popular video and radio programs under the Doom and Bloom™ label.

THE ALTONS' MISSION

To put a medically-prepared person in every family for any disaster. A family that prepares will have the best chance to succeed, even if everything else fails.

PREFACE

+++

A DIFFERENT KIND OF MEDICAL BOOK

During my youth, I was privileged to serve as a resident in Miami's large inner-city hospital and, later, as a private practitioner in a middle-class suburban area. In every sense of the word, my experience was conventional: standard medical training, easy access to modern supplies, and only a few minutes wait to transport a patient to an advanced critical care center.

Even when I volunteered to help as Hurricane Andrew ravaged parts of South Florida in 1992, the victims I encountered were never truly beyond access to help. Emergency personnel were there; some, like myself, were present during the storm itself. Yet, even in an age where the ambulance is just minutes away, disasters happen that eliminate access to the miracle of modern medicine. We are thrown back, at least temporarily, to an earlier era.

The thought of losing access to medical care is hard to accept for the average citizen. After all, they have enjoyed its benefits their entire lives. With decades of peace and relative prosperity, most in developed countries cannot fathom how such a scenario can occur. The end result is that we have lost the resiliency needed in times of adversity.

Many of the skills our ancestors learned have not been passed on to recent generations. Few families remember any of the natural remedies commonly used by their own grandparents. They value a well-manicured lawn more than a healthy medicinal herb garden.

We live in an age of treatment standards and protocols. They exist for a reason and most benefit the patient population. Although well-documented to save lives, they are often rigid and without variation. Any divergence from the conventional wisdom is met with criticism.

These days, most medical personnel specialize in a particular field. It's hard to blame them; certainly, there's a lot to know. An orthopedic surgeon is unlikely to be an expert in treating heart disease. A midwife probably doesn't know how to pull teeth. A paramedic may be comfortable with trauma and other emergencies, but not the long-term management of diabetes.

This trend to specialize has led to an erosion in the ability of healthcare providers to function as general practitioners. Indeed, there is such a shortage of "family doctors" that incentives are offered to those willing to go into the field.

Thus, many physicians spend their careers reading x-rays, treating cancer or performing cardiac bypasses. These are certainly important skills, but how does such a person deal with the basic medical problems of trauma and infection you'd see in the aftermath of a long-term disaster?

The issue is compounded if you remove access to lab studies and high-tech diagnostics. The truth is that, as a society, we have failed to instill a culture of preparedness into, not only medical personnel, but the average citizen. The result of this failure leaves us less competent to deal with the ramifications of major "knock-you-off-the-power-grid" catastrophes.

Hurricane Katrina in 2005 serves as a perfect example of what happens when citizens and medical personnel are robbed of their access to medical technology and facilities. Flooding made it difficult for assistance teams to reach some who desperately needed help. The sheer number of people who required medical aid overwhelmed, at least in the early going, the resources available.

This event made us realize there are circumstances where the average person may wind up being the highest medical asset left to their people. Our mission became to place a medically prepared person in every family. In addition, we wanted to encourage medical professionals to consider what they would do if modern medicine became inaccessible.

To achieve these goals, we've spent a decade writing about what to do to keep people healthy in austere settings. This often involved educating them in the use of supplies for which they had limited or no training. It also meant teaching prevention, which, truly, is worth a hundred cures.

At times, it required designing a plan of action to treat disease and injury in the absence of lab tests, X-rays, and today's modern technology. All of this education was aimed at empowering the average citizen to save lives in disasters.

We faced hard realities in these efforts. There were times we realized that a medical problem would be beyond the ability of a caregiver without modern drugs and diagnostic equipment. Many strategies we formulated, including some here, couldn't hold a candle to today's medical marvels.

Why this book, then? We thought about what would cause the greatest number of illnesses and, perhaps, avoidable deaths in a long-term disaster scenario. We realized that infection would be a major scourge in situations where modern medicine was inaccessible. Just drinking questionable water could lead to diseases like dysentery and others that caused innumerable deaths in the past. During the Civil War, more soldiers died from complications of infectious illnesses than bullets or shrapnel.

Our research on this subject has led us to write this book about infectious diseases and antibiotics. Although antibiotics have been in common use since the second World War, they are not available to the average citizen without prescription.

In normal times, this is a very good thing: We are experiencing an epidemic of bacterial resistance due to overuse, not only by medical providers, but by agri-business in food-producing livestock. If we lose the grid due to a long-term disaster, however, the judicious use of antibiotics by the family medic might mean the difference between life and death.

This book is a primer on the infectious diseases most likely to rear their ugly heads in such scenarios. In it, you will find information regarding many of those diseases, the bacterial culprits involved, and the drugs used to treat them. This includes reasons to use or not use these medicines, how much to use for different ailments, the risks associated, and more.

We have been criticized for making this information available. Indeed, we admit that some of it is well beyond the conventional medical wisdom.

Much is hypothetical in nature, taking lessons learned from disasters in underdeveloped nations and extrapolating the effects to an advanced society. There are few examples of the complete loss of medical infrastructure in a 21st century nation; we can only theorize what the plan of action should be in, say, Chicago if an infectious disease outbreak occurred during a long-term power blackout.

Thinking about strategies to help the medically-responsible in such catastrophes, however, may prevent loss of life. Our goal is to instill a culture of medical preparedness in our readers; to develop a multitude of medics held in reserve for major calamities in the uncertain future. With thousands of such medically prepared people at the ready, citizens will survive who otherwise might not.

The sheer number of bacterial infections and the drugs used to treat them are too many to consider this book a complete review. Rather, basics of a number of common as well as serious infections are discussed in some detail. Many of these diseases are problems now; others were once a scourge but may return if we lose access to modern care.

The antibiotics discussed in this book are specifically those that, at present, are easily available for the general public to accumulate for disaster medical storage.

This book is not an academic textbook. Nor is it a guidebook on how to survive a zombie apocalypse. It is a collection of our thoughts, in plain English, on infectious disease and antibiotic treatment. For those looking for a more detailed discussion on these and other off-grid medical topics, please consider a copy of our book **"The Survival Medicine Handbook: The Essential Guide for When Medical Help is Not on the Way."** "The Survival Medicine Handbook" covers over 150 different medical issues that may confront the medic in long-term disaster scenarios.

This book is also not a medical diploma. Readers should understand that the practice of medicine without a license is illegal and punishable by law. If there is an existing medical system with trained personnel available, seek it out.

If not, it is our responsibility as good citizens to do what we can to help. If we take that responsibility seriously, our society might keep it together, even if everything else falls apart.

JOSEPH ALTON MD
AMY ALTON ARNP

NOTE: This book is meant for the non-medically trained, so we have attempted to avoid using technical medical terms when possible. You will often find such words in bold letters (for example, **"antibiotics" or "austere")** and defined in the glossary section.

INTRODUCTION

✚✚✚

A WAR OF WORLDS

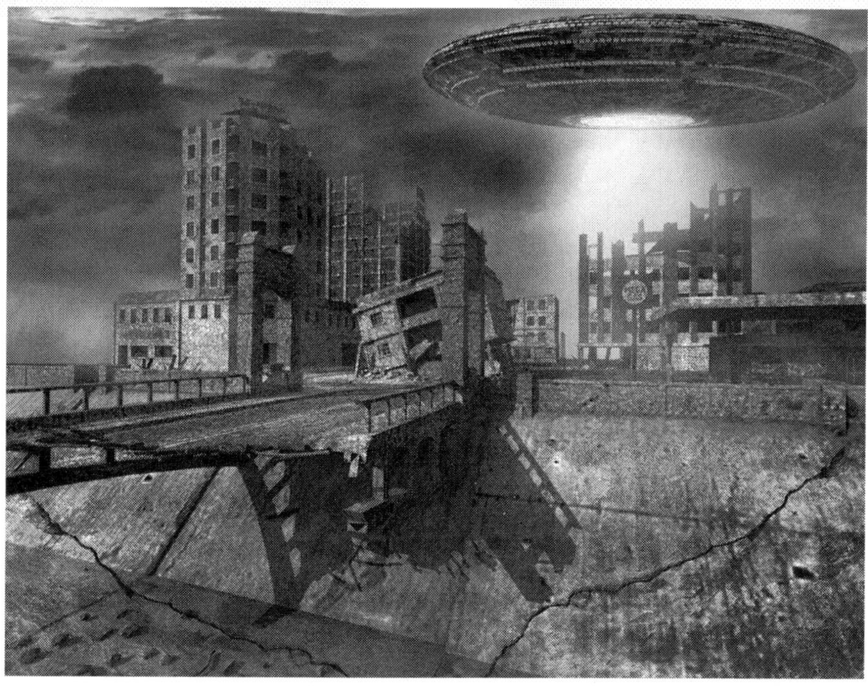

In 1938's "War of the Worlds," a radio broadcast that became a hit movie, an invasion force from Mars attacks the Earth. As the Martians lay waste to the entire planet, no weapon wielded by man can stop the imminent destruction of human civilization. Only when a bacterial infection takes root in the Martian force does the onslaught finally cease. The aliens, it seems, had no natural resistance to Earth's tiniest inhabitants; the invaders were annihilated in short order.

Leaving the realm of science fiction, there are many instances where even the strongest creatures on Earth fall victim to bacteria. We read recently about the death of Tilikum, a killer whale at the Sea World Marine park in Orlando, Florida. You may remember him from the movie "Blackfish."

Like many large animals forced to live a cramped existence, Tilikum was subject to both physical and mental stress. In 2017, the powerful 22 foot-long, 12,500-pound whale died as a result of a bacterial lung infection. His mass and strength could not overcome an invasion by one-celled microbes invisible to the naked eye.

Just as bacteria destroyed the Martians in "War of the Worlds" and Tilikum at Sea World, infection can snuff out the lives of the healthiest human Earthlings. A war of worlds, the microscopic against the macroscopic, has been raging for thousands of years.

Even in modern times, large numbers of people are killed annually by disease-causing germs. Although this happens most often in less developed countries, don't think that affluent countries are immune: Cases of exotic infections, some resistant to every known treatment, can be found in the most advanced medical facilities.

What Is Infection?

Everyone has heard of the word and the tools that physicians use to treat them, but what, really, is infection? **Infection** is the invasion of a living being by a **pathogen**, an organism which can cause disease. These organisms, usually too small to be seen with the naked eye, invade the body in different ways. They multiply and cause effects on their "**hosts**" which are detrimental to health.

The actions of a pathogen are opposed to those of what we call "**normal flora**." Normal flora consists of bacteria in or on our bodies that do not cause disease.

An infection may be "**subclinical**" and reveal no evidence of its presence for the time being, or it may be "**clinical**" and show obvious signs and symptoms. An infection may be "**localized**" and stay in one area or organ, or it may be "**systemic**" and spread through the entire body. The end result, if untreated, may be life-threatening.

Pathogens include various types of **bacteria, viruses, protozoa,** and **fungi**. The species that can produce ill effects in humans are numerous, but not all microorganisms cause disease; indeed, most are perfectly harmless. Others are beneficial, such as certain gut bacteria necessary for the proper digestion of food. When a microorganism lives on a host without any ill effect, it is called a "**colonization**" rather than an infection.

Although it's true that most microbes are benign, some are downright deadly, like the Ebola virus or the bacteria that causes Pneumonic Plague. These pathogens may arrive in a community unexpectedly in sudden outbreaks or, like malaria in tropical nations, may represent a constant threat throughout the year. In addition, diseases new to an area or new to science altogether are constantly emerging.

Antibiotics: Both Sides of the Coin

A number of infectious diseases, mostly respiratory and intestinal, consistently rank in the top ten causes of global deaths every year. Therefore, it can be argued that the development of antibiotics is one of the most important advances in medicine over the last century. These drugs have turned millions of what were once inevitable deaths into avoidable ones.

Yet, like most medical marvels, there is another side to the coin. Overuse of antibiotics, especially in food-producing livestock, has caused many bacteria to exhibit resistance to these drugs. Some pathogens have mutated to become impervious to all known medications and, despite constant efforts to develop new antibiotics, the increase in numbers of resistant bacteria outpaces the research.

Therefore, it is important to use antibiotics wisely. Antibiotic treatment is the domain of medical professionals, but under what circumstances would it be appropriate to use antibiotics if you're not a physician? Few and far between, we would think; but when the ambulance isn't just around the corner, someone has to take responsibility for keeping people safe.

You might find such a scenario hard to imagine. In a major disaster, however, the sheer number of casualties might make it difficult for the ill and injured to get the medical care they needed. The 2011 earthquake in Haiti is a classic example of the demand for medical care overwhelming the available resources.

There are many other examples where help may not be on the way. In a backcountry expedition, ocean voyage, or any other austere setting, emergency services may not be accessible. A remote homestead or a mission overseas may mean that, for the time being, the average citizen becomes their family's highest medical asset.

Of course, if there is a functioning modern medical system where you are, seek it out. In short term events, medical help is likely already on the way, and the possibility of a bad outcome is small. In longer-term events, however, the risk associated with an infection that is ignored for weeks is great. The end result may be tragic. Therefore, knowledge and training are important for those thrust into the role of healthcare providers in the aftermath of a catastrophe.

All the tools available must be utilized. Healers of old based their treatments on observations regarding the effects of certain herbs. This led to an entire discipline called **herbalism**, which, at the time, constituted the majority of conventional medical practice. Since then, modern drugs like antibiotics have revolutionized the practice of medicine.

If the family medic is armed with a way to fight infection, the chance for success increases, even if everything else fails. This is why obtaining antibiotics for your disaster medical storage is incredibly important.

Having said that, the notion of a non-medical person having antibiotics on hand in disaster settings is frowned upon by the conventional medical wisdom, and for good reason. Yet, if a family member is dying of an infection and there is no ambulance coming to render aid or hospital to treat the patient, the average citizen may need to act. Learning about infections and the medicines that treat them is a prerequisite for the effective "**medic**" in austere scenarios.

Here's the reason why: In the history channel film "**After Armageddon**," a paramedic takes his family on the road after an apocalyptic event. During their travels, they meet a community that can use someone with medical training and join it to start a new life.

All hands are needed, however, to grow food and perform other activities of daily survival. Our hero is assigned to duties to which he is not accustomed. He ends up with a minor injury that soon becomes infected. Unfortunately, the medical supplies of the community are limited; they ran out of **anti-biotics** long ago. He watches his infection spread over the next few weeks; despite his extensive knowledge and training, it eventually kills him. If antibiotics had been available, the final outcome could have been quite different.

This scenario could repeat itself thousands of times in a major long-term disaster. This book is our attempt to prevent avoidable deaths in any situation where modern medical care is not accessible. In it, the average person will learn the basics of infectious disease and the substances that treat it. By absorbing the information plainly presented here, family medics will be more effective in keeping their loved ones healthy during emergencies.

Note that we often mention "the average person" or "the family medic." The truth is that board-certified microbiologists and many other medical professionals will find this book below their pay grade. This book isn't a college textbook. It is meant to help educate non-medical personnel in a practical, no-frills manner.

The Austere Medic

In our research, we take the experience of those in remote locations with limited supplies as guidance. The experiences of people like medical missionaries identify likely health issues that would occur in austere settings. It wasn't unusual to see the following:

Trauma

- Minor musculoskeletal injuries (sprains and strains)
- Minor trauma (cuts, scrapes)
- Major traumatic injury (fractures, occasional knife and/or gunshot wounds)
- Burn injuries (all degrees)

Infection

- Respiratory infections (pneumonia, bronchitis, influenza, common colds)
- Diarrheal disease (sometimes a community-wide outbreak)
- Infected wounds
- Minor infections (for example, urinary infections, "pinkeye")
- Sexually transmitted diseases
- Lice, ticks, mosquitos, and the diseases they carry

Allergic reactions

- Minor (bees, bed bugs, or other insect bites and stings)
- Major (anaphylactic shock)

Dental

- Toothaches
- Broken or knocked-out teeth
- Loss fillings
- Loose crowns or other dental work

Women's' Issues

- Pregnancy
- Miscarriage
- Childbirth

The above was published in our book "**The Survival Medicine Handbook: The Essential Guide for When Medical Help is Not on the Way.**" When we took a second look at the list, we realized that almost every medical issue was either infectious in nature or could be complicated by infection. It stands to reason, therefore, that a medic without an understanding of how to identify and treat infectious disease is unlikely to be of much help in a long-term disaster.

Although the reader will gain insight into many diseases and the drugs used to treat them, it is important to realize that the best a caregiver, even that board-certified microbiologist, can achieve without advanced lab studies is a series of educated guesses:

- What is the disease?
- Are bacteria causing it?
- Which one is responsible? Is an antibiotic needed?
- Which antibiotic will be most effective against the offending organism?

It's quite a challenge, but if lives are to be saved, one that must be accepted. By making a series of logical decisions, the family medic will be more likely to make the diagnosis. More information means a better chance to keep their loved ones healthy in emergencies.

The words of President Theodore Roosevelt should echo in the mind of every person responsible for the health of their people in difficult times: **"Do what you can, with what you have, where you are."**

NOTE: This book is meant for the non-medically trained, so we have attempted to avoid using technical medical terms when possible. Words in bold letters (for example, "**antibiotics**" or "**austere**") are defined in the glossary section.

TABLE OF CONTENTS

SECTION 1

INFECTIOUS DISEASE

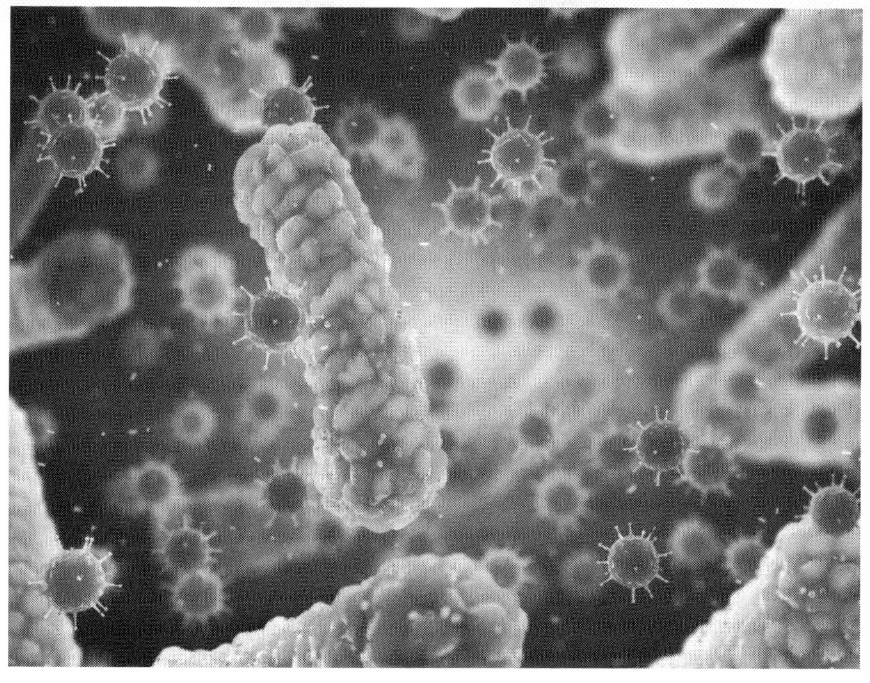

PATHOGENS (DISEASE-CAUSING ORGANISMS)

In order to understand the use of antibiotics in infectious disease, we must first understand infectious disease. To understand infectious disease, we must first understand the organisms that cause it.

As mentioned in the introduction, a pathogen is an organism that has the ability to damage a host when it invades. In its broadest sense, the definition includes any agent that can cause disease, but the term is usually used to describe a microbe.

Microscopic germs cause injury to tissues in a number of ways. They may produce toxic substances that damage organs or interfere with vital cell processes like reproduction. They may invade host tissues and consume them. Their presence may cause damage by triggering the human immune system to over-respond.

First, however, they must enter the body. Invasion may be direct or involve a "middle-man" known as a "vector." "Vectors," from the Latin word meaning "one who carries," carry and transmit a pathogen to others. They may be another human, an animal, or even a microbe.

A vector does not have to be ill themselves. A mosquito, for example, carries the parasite that causes malaria in humans but doesn't experience the disease. Ticks carry the bacteria that causes Lyme disease without any ill effect whatsoever.

Another example of a disease vector was a domestic servant known as "Typhoid Mary" Mallon. From 1900-1907, she worked as a cook for various families in New York City. She was a carrier of the pathogen for Typhoid fever, which she transmitted to at least 50 people without feeling sick herself.

The elimination of a vector from the environment (terminating Mary's employment, for example) usually ends the outbreak of disease. This is exactly what happened when Mary Mallon was identified as the vector and quarantined for three years. When she returned to work as a cook for a women's hospital in 1915, however, she caused a second outbreak that sickened 25 people.

TYPES OF PATHOGENS

Bacteria

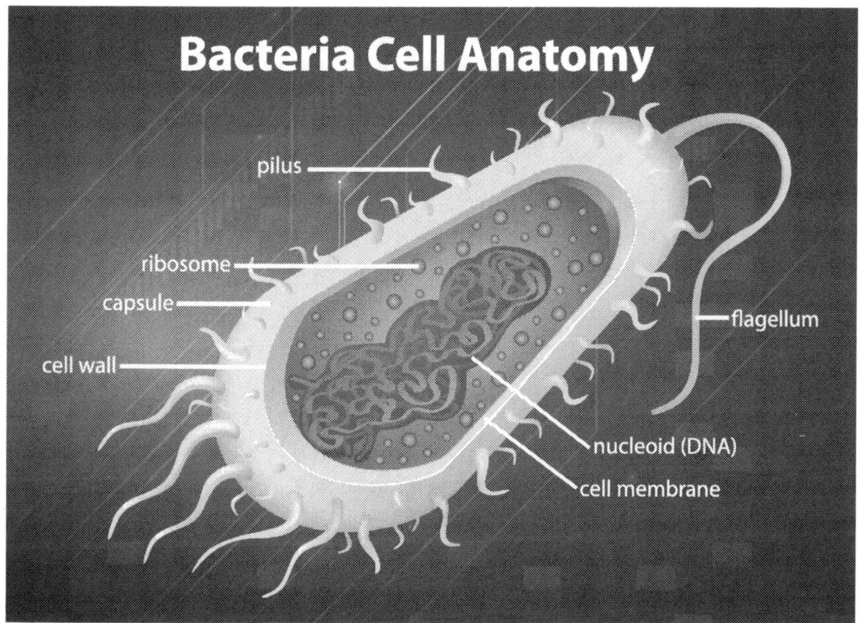

There are a number of different pathogens that cause infectious disease. Bacterial infection is the focus of this book since it is the organism most likely to be affected by antibiotics. First, note that the word "bacteria" is the plural form. A single one is called a "**bacterium.**"

Bacteria were among the first life forms on Earth but are alien to humans in many ways. They are **prokaryotes**, one-celled organisms so simple that they have no **nucleus** and but a single **chromosome** to hold genetic material;

Humans, animals, and plants are eukaryotes. Each cell of a **eukaryote**, whether a microscopic parasite or a blue whale, is structurally more complex than a bacterium.

Despite their simplicity, bacteria contain a well-developed cell structure with **"organelles"** unique to them alone. These include **"ribosomes"** that make proteins and **"plasmids"** that contain genetic material used for special purposes. All of these are enveloped by a cell membrane.

Bacteria are present everywhere. They inhabit the soil in your backyard. They live at the bottom of the ocean and in Antarctic wastelands. Bacteria exist (most likely) as far away as Mars and as close as the inside of your body. In fact, just one gram of your feces contains about one trillion of them! If you took the population of bacteria on Earth, they would far outnumber the entire plant and animal population combined.

Given that fact, it's fortunate that most bacteria are completely harmless. Some, however, can cause seriously dangerous infectious diseases, including cholera, syphilis, anthrax, leprosy, and bubonic plague.

Bacteria obtain nourishment in various ways. Some have the ability to use photosynthesis like plants do. Others can break down organic or inorganic substances in their environment. Those that have the most connection with humans interact with them in one of three ways:

- **Commensalistic:** Bacteria benefit without an appreciable effect on humans. For example, bacteria on our skin obtain nourishment by eating dead cells. Humans neither benefit nor suffer as a result.
- **Mutualistic:** Both bacteria and humans benefit. For example, intestinal bacteria allow us to digest food; in return, they obtain food as well.
- **Parasitic:** Bacteria benefit at the expense of humans. For example, cholera bacteria reproduce in human hosts, causing dire consequences like severe diarrhea, dehydration, and even death.

Bacteria come in a variety of shapes, ranging from spheres to rods to spirals. Many have a mode of locomotion in the form of a tail-like appendage called a "**flagellum**." Others have hair-like structures on the outside called "**pili**" that help them attach to other cells.

Bacteria even have a unique way of reproducing: During growth, they make a copy of their genetic material and organelles. Once reaching a certain size, a bacterium splits into two "daughter" cells via a process called "**binary fission**."

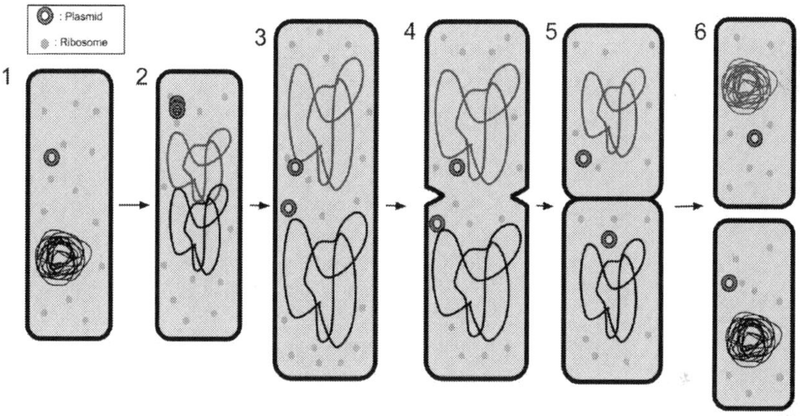

Bacterial Reproduction by Binary Fission

There are many different species of bacteria. Most bacteria don't need to enter the host's cells to reproduce. They do just fine, for example, in your blood. A subgroup of bacteria called **Rickettsia**, however, does require entry, growth, and reproduction within a host cell.

Rickettsiae are the cause of typhus, Rocky Mountain spotted fever, and a number of other infectious diseases. Despite the name, Rickettsia do not cause "**rickets**." Rickets is a deformity of long bones in young children which is a result of vitamin D deficiency.

The grand majority of bacterial infections are treatable with **antibiotics**. These drugs can be life-saving but they can also be life-threatening if not used wisely. This subject is covered in detail later in this book.

Viruses

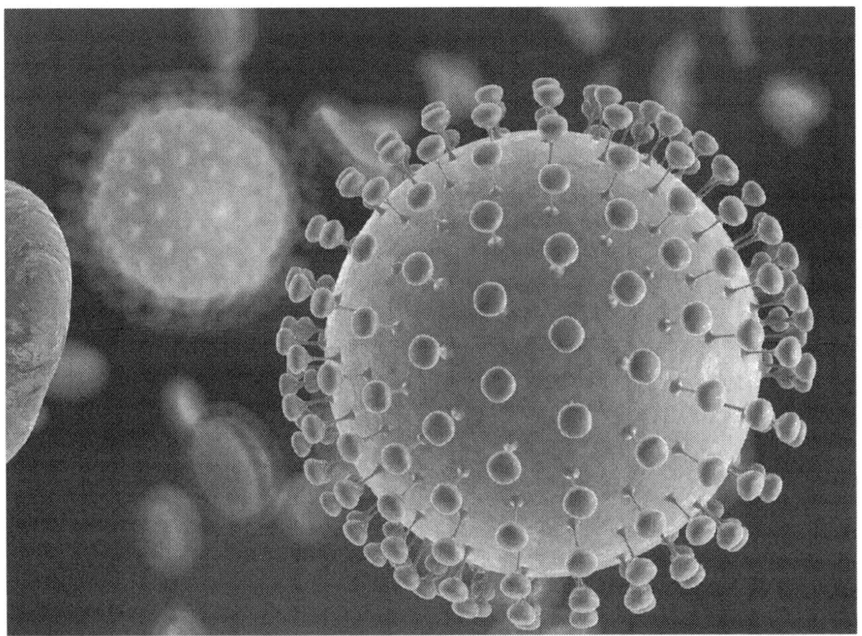

Viruses are microscopic pathogens that, unlike most bacteria, can reproduce only inside the living cells of other organisms. Viruses are very simple entities that rarely consist of much more than a bit of genetic code covered by a protein coat (a "**capsid**").

This simplicity doesn't mean that viruses are harmless. The very dangerous Ebola virus, for example, is thought to have a total of 7 genes and no chromosomes. Human beings, on the other hand, have around 20,000 genes crowded into 23 chromosomes.

Viruses don't eat or grow; in truth, they stretch the very definition of life. A viral particle without a host is known as a "**virion**"; it only acts as a living organism when it enters a host cell.

Viruses can reproduce like living things, but not without the host's help. The process of viral reproduction occurs as follows:

- The virus finds a host cell and binds to it.
- The virus injects its genetic material into the host cell.
- The genetic material replicates using the host's cellular machinery.
- New viruses are produced within the host.
- New viruses are expelled from the host cell (killing it).

Viruses can infect all types of hosts, from animals and plants all the way down to bacteria. Examples of human diseases caused by viruses include the common cold, influenza, chickenpox, rabies, hepatitis, herpes, Ebola, and Zika.

Like other pathogens, viruses can be spread by:

- Mosquitoes and other **vectors**
- Airborne droplets in coughs or sneezes
- Contact with blood or other bodily fluids
- Ingestion of contaminated food or water

A normal immune system can often kill the infecting virus. However, some viruses evade these immune responses and result in chronic infections, such as HIV or Hepatitis C.

New pandemic-level viruses have emerged in the 21st century that have killed millions and infected hundreds of millions. Although this book is specifically focused on bacterial infections and the antibiotics that treat them, consider the book "Alton's Pandemic Preparedness Guide" for much more on viral diseases.

Bacterial vs. Viral Anatomy

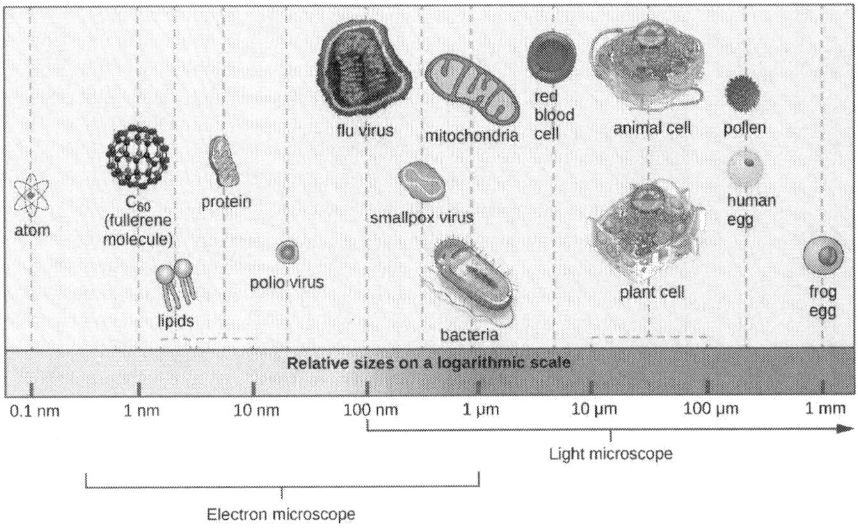

Bacteria and viruses are the two pathogens of most concern to health departments in the United States. Although both can be **virulent** (capable of causing disease), they are quite different from each other:

Bacteria are:

- 10-100 times larger than viruses
- Structurally more complex
- Capable of reproducing on their own; viruses need a host to multiply.
- Intercellular organisms (most live between cells; viruses invade cells (Intracellular).

Although some are resistant, bacteria are generally susceptible to standard antibiotic therapy as it is used today. On the other hand, viruses are immune to the effect of these drugs. We are in the infancy of antiviral research; there are antiviral drugs on the market today, but most are limited in their action and effectiveness.

Protozoa

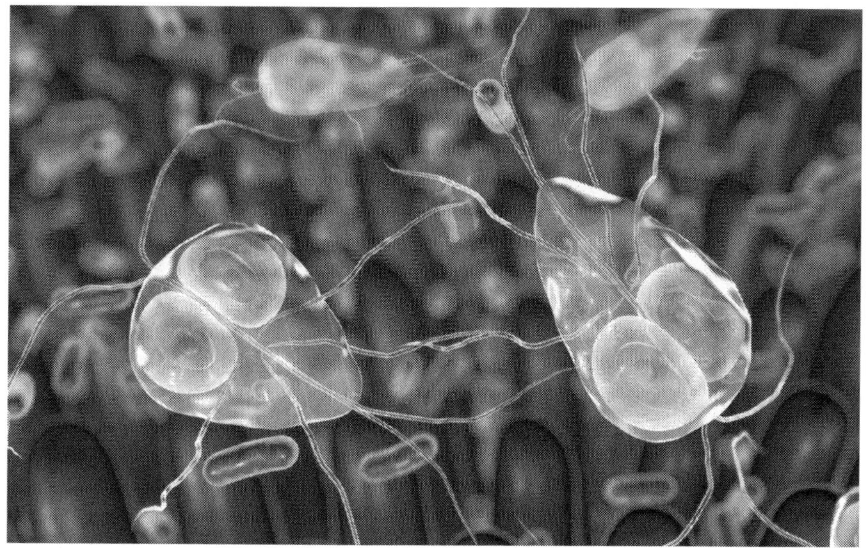

Protozoa, a member of the **protist** "kingdom" of life, are one-celled microbes that represent a step up the ladder. Unlike bacteria, these one-celled organisms are **eukaryotes**. Although protozoans are comprised of one cell, they have a nucleus and more specialized **organelles** than **prokaryotes** like bacteria.

Protozoa were once considered unicellular "animals" because they prey on microbes and exhibit other behaviors seen in higher life forms. In fact, they are more closely related to humans than bacteria.

Some differences between protozoa and bacteria include size and method of obtaining energy. Bacteria are generally smaller than protozoa. Protozoa "eat" by enveloping their prey (often, bacteria); bacteria simply absorb nutrients through their cell walls.

Protozoa are most commonly found in aquatic environments, although some can be found in moist soils or mosses. Bacteria are everywhere. Like bacteria, many protists have tail-like appendages called **flagella** that they whip around for locomotion.

Transmission of both protozoal or bacterial disease to humans commonly occurs by drinking contaminated water. Either of these microbes, however, may be spread by animal vectors.

Although protozoa need a moist habitat, some can form inactive drought-resistant forms known as "**cysts**"; they can remain dormant for periods of time until conditions become more favorable. The actively feeding form is known as a "**trophozoite**" and is responsible for ill effects on humans.

Protozoa cause infectious diseases in humans such as malaria, giardia, some dysenteries, sleeping sickness, and amoebiasis. A common sexually-transmitted vaginal infection is caused by a protozoan called *trichomonas.*

Unlike viruses, protozoa are usually susceptible to treatment with certain antibiotics.

Fungi

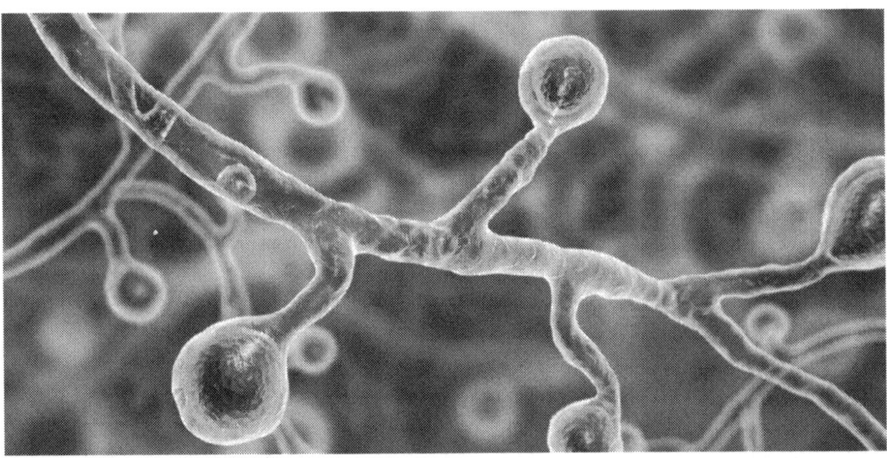

Fungi (singular form: fungus) are **eukaryotic.** They include one-celled microorganisms known as yeasts but also multi-celled entities like mushrooms and molds. Fungi are not plants; they contain no mechanism to use **photosynthesis** to make energy. Instead, they absorb decaying matter in their environment.

Fungi are composed of filaments called **hyphae**; their cells are thread-like and usually connect end-to-end to each other. An aggregate of hyphae is known as a "**mycelium**" and is considered a single organism. Fungal colonies composed of **mycelia** are found in or on soil and many other places.

An interesting feature of fungi is the presence of a substance called "**chitin**" in their cell walls. This is a fibrous carbohydrate that also exists in the exoskeletons of insects, spiders, and crustaceans. Chitin gives structural support to fungal cells.

Unless they are visible as mushrooms or molds, fungi act microscopically to decompose organic matter in areas like the forest floor. Thus, they have a vital ecological role in cycling nutrients. Fungi aid humans by acting as a fermenting agent, an ingredient for making bread, or a direct food source. More recently, they have been used to help produce many of the antibiotics we'll discuss in this book, including penicillin.

Although beneficial in that sense, infections with fungi can range from a minor annoyance to a life-threatening disease. Areas you'll see most commonly affected are the skin and mucous membranes like the oral cavity and vagina. In those with weakened immune systems, however, any organ is susceptible. They are treated with anti-fungal medications in topical or oral form.

Helminths

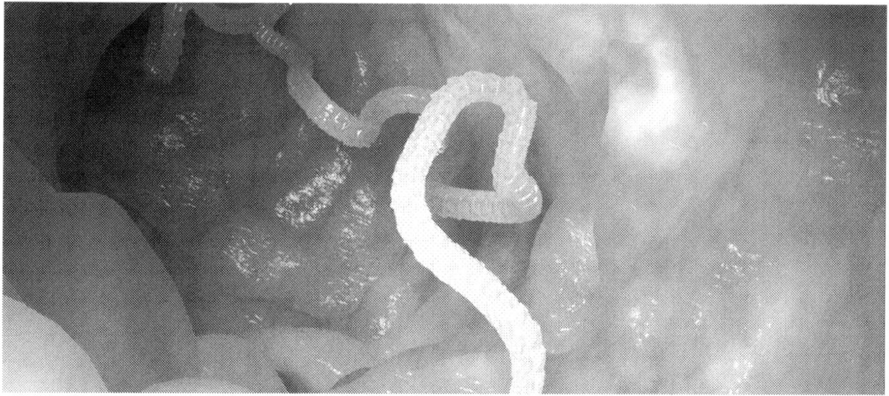

Although we consider infections as caused by microscopic organisms, some are caused by multi-celled parasites that can be quite large. The word "**parasite**" comes from the Greek word "parastos," meaning "someone that eats at someone else's table." A significant portion of the world's population is infected with these organisms.

Intestinal worms or "**helminths**" are parasites that invade the human body and derive nutrition from the human gut. They are **endoparasites** that live deep in our intestines or other core organs, often gaining sustenance by sharing our partly-digested food. Helminths are notorious egg-laying machines, with some depositing tens of thousands a day into their host.

Most helminths are found in the soil. According to the Centers for Disease Control and Prevention, the three most common parasitic worm infections are:

- **Ascaris**: close to one billion cases
- **Whipworms**: 600-800 million cases
- **Hookworms**: 576-740 million cases

In the United States and Canada, **pinworms** are the most common helminthic infection.

The grand majority of victims are found in underdeveloped countries where sanitation is questionable and human feces contaminate the soil. Helminth eggs enter the body when hands and bare feet touch egg-laden soil or a person consumes vegetables or fruit that have not been properly washed. Once ingested, the eggs hatch with the help of stomach acid and the worms take up residence in the gut. One variety known as "hookworms" can also enter the body by penetrating bare skin that comes in contact with the soil.

Parasitic worms may also enter the body through poorly or unevenly cooked food. **Trichinosis** is an infection caused by the roundworm *Trichinella* in undercooked pork. One or two days after exposure, trichinosis causes diarrhea and other intestinal symptoms along with fever, headache, muscle pain, and swelling around the eyes.

Some worms can reach impressive lengths in the human body. Tapeworms, for example, have been reported to reach a length of 80 feet in the intestines. Others, like pinworms, remain microscopic.

Drugs that eliminate worm infections (sometimes called **infestations**) include the prescription medicines Mebendazole and Albendazole. These are commonly referred to as "**anti-helminthics**" as opposed to antibiotics.

THE HISTORY OF BACTERIA

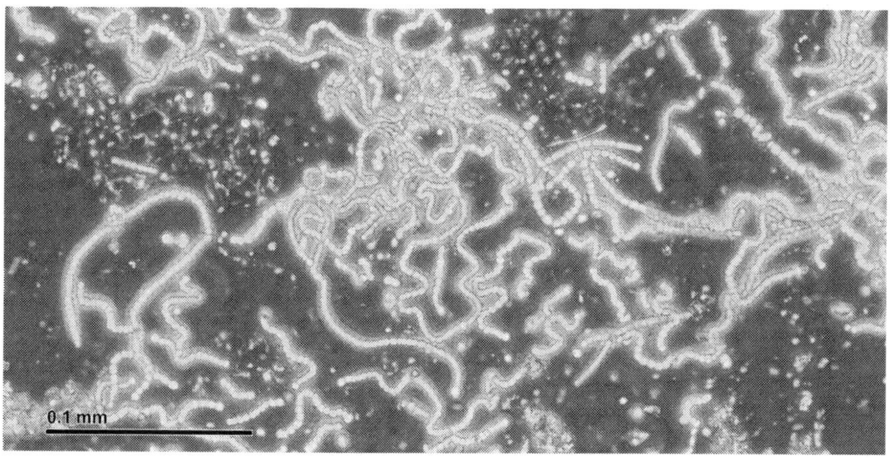

Cyanobacteria were the first life forms on Earth

To better understand current events, it's useful to know the history behind them. The same can be said of the developments through time that led humans to learn about bacteria.

Bacteria have played their part in the evolution of the planet for eons. Fossils of microorganisms have been discovered in stone dating more than 400 million years old. Some argue that primitive bacteria existed almost as far back as the very beginning of Earth's history. For the majority of their time on Earth, they were the predominant life form and left their mark, good and bad, on every species that came after them.

The presence of oxygen in the atmosphere and, thus, the possibility of life as we know it, is a consequence of bacteria; specifically, **cyanobacteria** (sometimes confusingly called, "blue-green algae"). Cyanobacteria were early users of a process called **photosynthesis**, where water, carbon dioxide, and sunlight combine to produce oxygen. Even today, the part of a plant cell which conducts photosynthesis (called a "**chloroplast**") is essentially a cyanobacterium.

Despite this, humans had little idea that bacteria were such a pervasive presence in our world. Indeed, we were completely unaware of their existence, if not the diseases they caused. As new innovations like magnifying glasses in the thirteenth century and simple microscopes in the sixteenth century were developed, we began to learn more about a world previously unknown.

It was not, however, until the invention of a more powerful microscope that bacteria were discovered. In 1676, Dutch "microscopist" Antonie van Leeuwenhoek was the first to publish articles on bacteria and protozoans (which he called "animalcules") as well as red blood cells and human sperm. Amazingly, his findings were considered mere curiosities, and there were no further reports on bacteria for a hundred years.

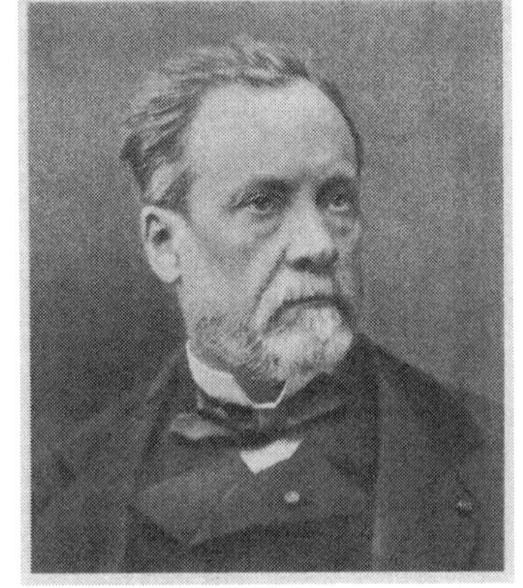

Louis Pasteur

By the mid-1800s, however, the connection between bacteria and disease was more fully appreciated as a result of the work of Louis Pasteur. He performed studies to determine why milk and wine went "sour" with time.

Pasteur concluded that bacteria were the culprits. He deduced that, if bacteria could make milk or wine "sick," then why not human beings? This assumption led to the **Germ Theory of Disease**, which suggested that microbes were the cause of infectious diseases.

Pasteur himself was unable to prove the theory, but a German scientist named Robert Koch performed an experiment that did. He injected mice with bacteria taken from animals that died from anthrax. The injected mice then all developed anthrax in short order.

It took the invention of the light bulb, patented in 1880 by Thomas Edison, for microscope technology to reach its maximum potential. Since then, various new techniques for visualizing microbes have been developed, such as **electron microscopy** and others. These greatly improved on the "light" microscope and afforded a more detailed look at bacteria and other microorganisms.

BACTERIAL CLASSIFICATION

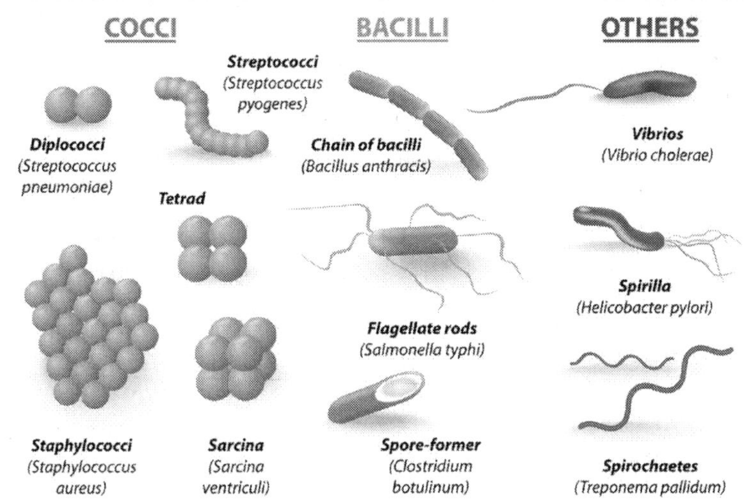

Once bacteria became visible through the microscope, efforts were made to classify the different types. Scientists found that bacteria came in various shapes, and made efforts to categorize them based upon their appearance. Bacteria may exist as:

Cocci: These bacteria are round or oval shaped. They may exist as individual entities, or may combine in different ways. A *monococcus* is what we call those cocci that remain apart from others of their species. A *diplococcus* consists of pairs of these cells. A *tetracoccus* aggregates into four round cells. *Staphylococcus* forms a cluster of cells that appears something like grapes. A *streptococcus* is a round bacteria that, when it divides, it does so in a manner that forms a chain. Still another is *sarcina,* which consists of four cocci or multiples that form a cube-like structure.

Bacilli: Many bacteria are cylindrical in shape and often referred to by microbiologists as "rods." Most appear as single cells, but others (*diplobacilli*) may have two attached end-to-end. *Streptobacilli*, like streptococci, form chains. Another arrangement you might see is a palisade-like formation, vaguely reminiscent of an old-style picket fence. Still another is the *coccobacilli*, short, stumpy rods that appear like a hybrid of bacilli and cocci.

Spirilli: Another group of bacterial cells appear curved. The simplest form is *vibrio* which would remind you of the shape of a comma. Spirilla appears longer with a rigid spiral shape. A third type, known as a "spirochete," is even more elaborate and flexible in its spiral shape.

Filaments: Filamentous bacteria are reminiscent of angel hair pasta in their appearance. Known as a "**Mycelium**," it consists of branching threads called "**hyphae**" similar to what is seen in a fungus. They sometimes form clusters or networks which branch out.

Pleomorphs: These bacteria, when seen under the microscope, have all sorts of different shapes.

Others even include bacteria shaped like stars or rectangles!

The Gram Stain

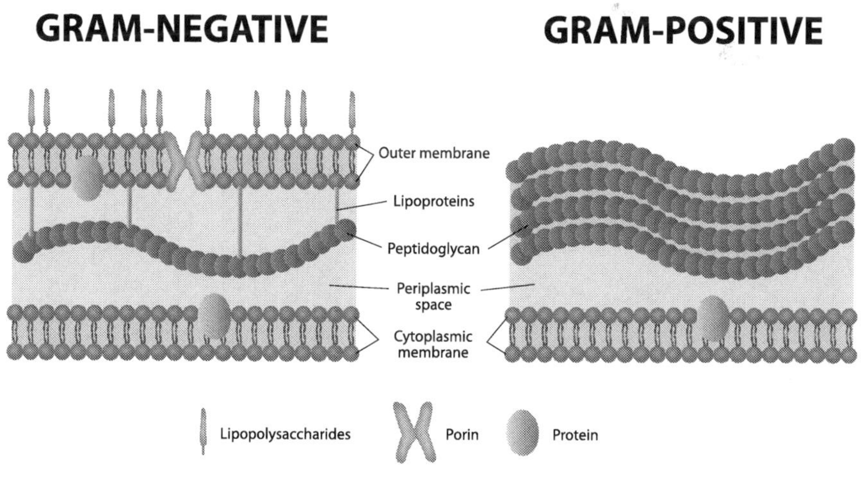

In the late 19th century, another technique for classifying bacteria was developed known as the **"Gram stain."** The name has nothing to do with the unit of weight; it was first formulated by the Danish scientist Hans Christian Gram.

Gram staining uses the effect of a certain dye called "crystal violet" on bacteria to classify different general types. Interestingly, the original intent by Gram was simply to make the organisms more clearly visible on microscopic examination.

The crystal violet dye stained some bacteria a purplish color. Adding a certain counterstain to the microscope slide colored many of the remaining bacteria pink. This method thus divided the microbes into two large groups Those that retained the violet dye were called **Gram-positive**; those stained pink were called **Gram-negative**.

Gram-positive bacteria have a thick cell wall made mostly (90%) of a substance called **peptidoglycan**. The more peptidoglycan, the more purple the appearance when exposed to crystal violet. Gram-negative bacteria have much less peptidoglycan, but are more chemically complex with an additional membrane and spaces between layers. These characteristics serve as a barrier to uptake of the violet dye. This is important because, for an antibiotic to work, it needs to be able to penetrate one or both bacterial cell wall types.

The Gram stain process is relatively simple:

- After heating the bacteria to "fix" them onto the microscope slide, the crystal violet dye is applied. (all organisms turn purple).
- Iodide is then added, which holds the violet dye in the cell.
- Alcohol or acetone is then added to the slide, which "decolorizes" all but Gram-positive bacteria.
- The slide is then counterstained with safranin or carbol fuchsin, turning Gram-negative bacteria pink.

Although this method didn't identify the exact *species* of bacteria, it later became useful when antibiotics were developed, as some drugs worked better on gram-positive organisms and others on gram-negative. The antibiotics that worked on only one type were termed "**narrow spectrum**," while those that killed or otherwise inhibited a wide variety of bacteria were known as "**broad spectrum**." The first antibiotics were mostly narrow spectrum, while later "generations" in, for example, the penicillin family, were broader spectrum in nature.

It should be noted that some microbes are "atypical" in that they seem to retain neither the dye nor the counterstain.

In the 20th century, microbiological **"cultures"** were developed. In a culture, bacteria-laden body fluid or other sample is applied to a plate known as a "petri dish." The plate has a substance called "agar" which encourage colonies of bacteria to grow. The colonies help identify the type of organism involved.

When small amounts of an antibiotic are added, the inhibition of colony growth is an indicator of its effectiveness against the organism. For example, if an antibiotic is added to a plate with bacteria, the area where the antibiotic was placed will be devoid of colonies *if* the bacteria is susceptible to the drug.

Modern research now allows the identification of bacteria by evaluating its DNA structure. Without advanced technology, however, cultures and DNA evaluations are unlikely to be available in grid-down settings. We will have to depend on physical signs and symptoms for **diagnosis**.

BASICS OF IMMUNITY

B-cell activation

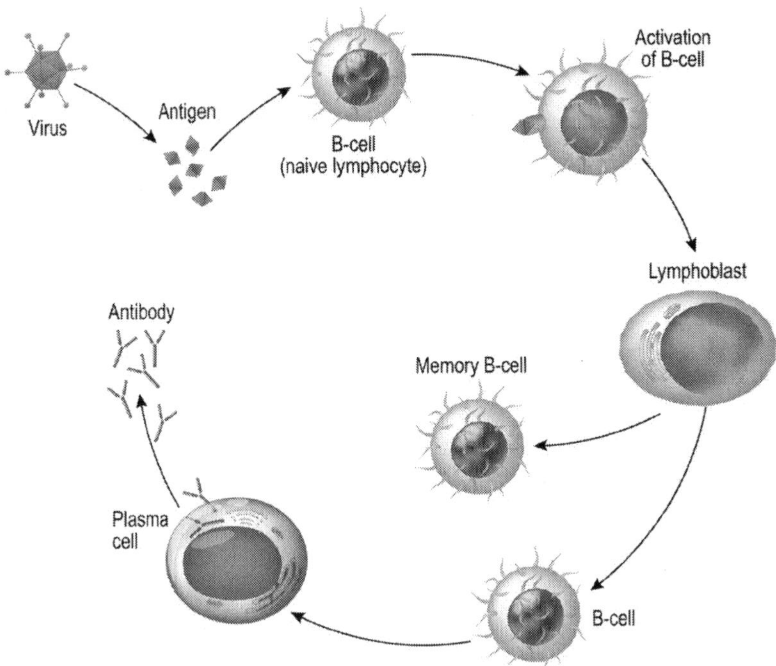

Our body is a fortress that is constantly under siege by bacteria, viruses, and other pathogens. Every day, we fight off attempts by one or another of these germs to gain a foothold.

Luckily, our immune system is usually aware of the presence of substances not recognizable as part of the body. The human response to infection involves the actions of certain cells and other substances called "**antibodies**" in blood.

Antibodies, B Cells, and T Cells

"**B lymphocytes**" produce specialized "**plasma cells**"; these, in turn, manufacture antibodies. Antibodies are Y-shaped proteins used by the immune system to pinpoint and eliminate pathogens. They are produced in quantity as a response to the presence of a toxin or other foreign product, also known as an "**antigen.**"

Resistance to an infection by the action of antibodies or white blood cells is known as "**immunity.**" One type of immune response is called "**humoral immunity**" (certain body fluids were once called "humours"). Humoral immunity involves the action of antibodies and works well to eliminate antigens found in blood.

Once a pathogen has invaded a cell, however, the antibodies can't see it and humoral immunity becomes ineffective. Another type, known as "**cell-mediated immunity,**" uses cells known as "**T-lymphocytes**" to identify and destroy cells that are infected.

Both B- and T-lymphocytes develop a subset of cells with a "memory" of the antigen they encountered. When they are exposed to the same antigen in the future, they mount a more rapid and stronger response against it.

Immunity can refer to resistance of an entire species or a particular individual to an illness (Typhoid Mary, for example, carried the typhoid germ without getting sick herself). Individual immunity is affected by many factors, such as age and genetics. Stress from nutritional deficiencies, environmental issues, or chronic illness may also play a role.

Categories of Immunity

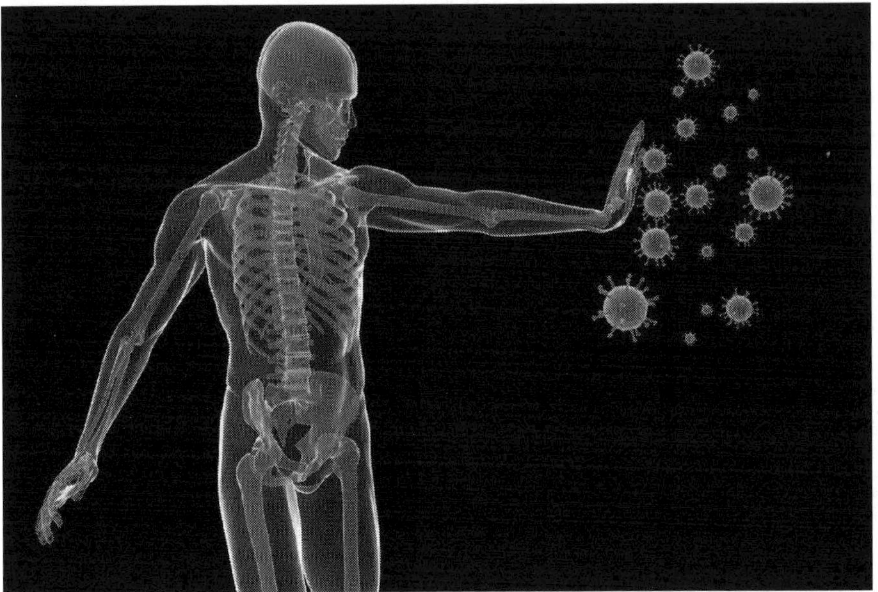

There are several categories of immunity that relate to infectious disease outbreaks:

Short-Term Immunity
Short-term immunity is the response we have when an infectious agent is detected, such as humoral or cell-mediated immunity. The body acts by producing a large amount of white blood cells like the T- and B-lymphocytes mentioned above. This initiates an immune response which attacks the invader. In newborns with immature immune systems, protection occurs as a result of breastfeeding. Antibodies may also be given by injection in certain cases.

During an **epidemic**, the population's ability to generate white cells increases its resistance. It is this property of the human body that causes the epidemic to eventually collapse.

Long-Term Immunity

The body's defenses retain a type of memory of the offending organism. If the pathogen returns to the area, that memory causes the body to produce a faster and stronger response against it. This is especially true with viral infections, such as "*Varicella*," a viral illness commonly known as 'chicken pox." Once you have had chicken pox, you are usually immune for the remainder of your life.

Natural Immunity

A particular individual, or occasionally an entire species, might possess the ability to resist a pathogen due to genetic factors passed on from generation to generation.

The Native American population of the New World had an extraordinarily high mortality rate when exposed to smallpox by the first European explorers. Those same explorers, however, had a much higher survival rate due to natural immunity bestowed upon them, generation after generation, by centuries of previous exposures.

Herd Immunity

When a large group (a "herd") possesses immunity, non-immune individuals within it enjoy a certain protection due to fewer exposures to an infection that may otherwise be fatal to them. The most common example today relates to vaccinated populations. If an unvaccinated person moves into an area where many are immune due to vaccinations, the likelihood of exposure drops significantly. This confers a certain level of protection. If many unvaccinated people move into an area, however, the overall "herd immunity" may be lost.

Vaccinations against influenza are usually made available to people in developed countries ahead of seasonal outbreaks in an effort to avoid infection. These are most effective if the flu virus is similar to last year's strain, as they use material from that virus to produce the vaccine. If the virus has mutated significantly, the vaccine may be ineffective. In one recent year, influenza vaccination conferred only 19% protection against the virus.

INFECTIOUS DISEASE OUTBREAKS

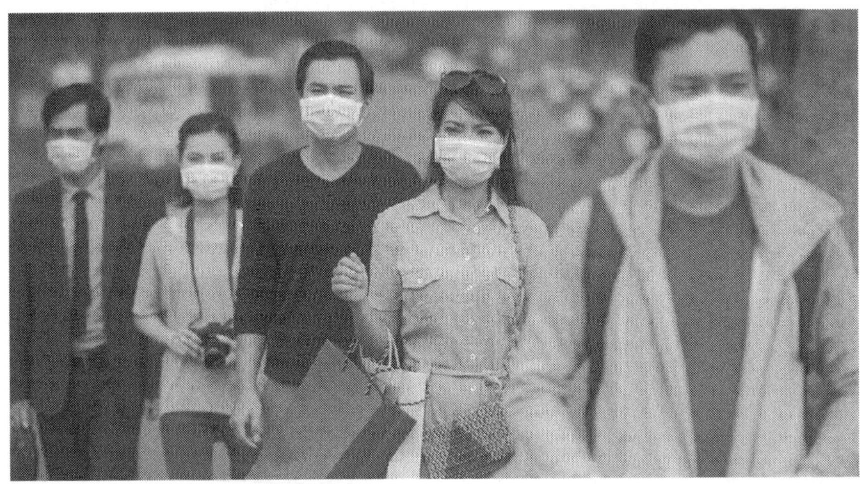

In modern times, we have become highly dependent on technology that has, in many cases, eliminated the scourge of infectious disease. Certain antibiotics are now available in their 3rd or 4th generation versions, and physicians aren't reluctant to use them when necessary.

Few, however, consider the possibility that a major disaster may wipe out the ability to manufacture these drugs in mass quantities. Severe restrictions exist which put these drugs out of the reach of the average person. What would happen if we are struck by a catastrophe that knocks out the power grid? We will be left with only the most basic options to deal with many medical issues.

Planning for disasters ahead of time will greatly increase your chances to avoid harm and stay safe. This is true for wildfires and floods, but it is also true for infectious disease outbreaks.

This book discusses the use of antibiotics in austere settings. Having antibiotics in your medical kit may be helpful for bacterial infections (but not the flu or other viruses). You can, however, minimize your chances of falling ill in any infectious disease outbreak with **non-pharmaceutical interventions** (NPIs). Consider the following NPI strategies:

- Stay home when you are sick or have been exposed to family members who are ill.
- Increase distance between people in settings where they commonly come into close contact with one another. This is known as "**social distancing**."
- Cover all coughs and sneezes with a tissue or, at least, your upper arm or elbow. Otherwise, germ-laden droplets can travel at least several feet; recent studies suggest even more dependent on the particle size.
- Wash hands or use hand sanitizer frequently.
- Cover your nose and mouth with a mask or cloth if you are sick and in the company of others.
- Clean all surfaces touched by sick people with a **disinfectant**.

NPIs are appropriate actions to take even if you are well-supplied with medications.

Endemic vs. Epidemic vs. Pandemic

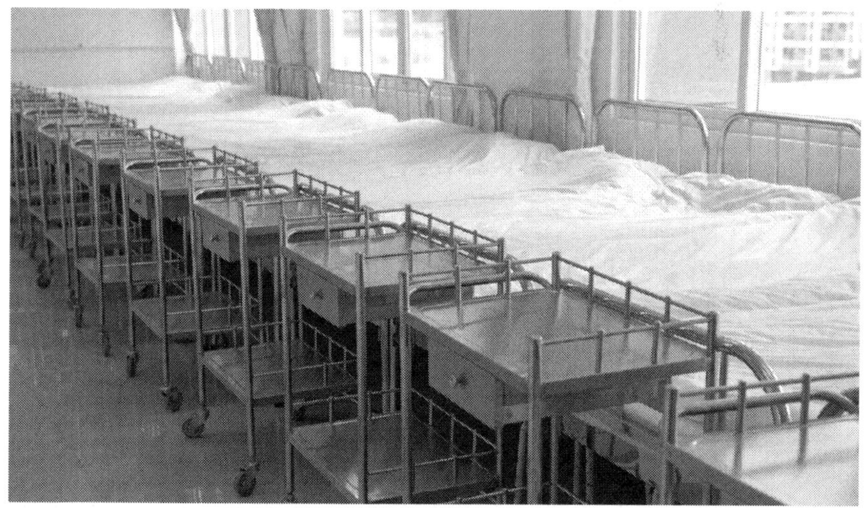

There may be instances where an infectious disease goes out of control. Everyone talks about epidemics and pandemics, but what are they? Let's start with some definitions so that you'll know what we're talking about:

An **Endemic** disease is a disease constantly found among a particular population or in a certain area. Malaria, for example, is endemic in many tropical countries. It is always there and cases are constantly being reported.

An **Epidemic** is a sudden and widespread outbreak of an infectious disease in a community that is not "endemic." Influenza is a good example of an epidemic disease: It arrives suddenly in seasonal waves, and is often at least slightly different genetically from its predecessors. Although it is still influenza, it may act more or less **virulent** based on how it has mutated.

A **Pandemic** occurs when an epidemic of infectious disease runs rampant throughout a large region or, in the case of the Great Spanish Flu Epidemic of 1918, the whole world.

World Health Organization Alerts For Outbreaks

The World Health Organization rates its level of concern about a disease entering a new area with Phase Alerts. The more severe the outbreak and perceived risk to humans, the higher the alert:

- **Phase 1:** The disease is found in animals; no known infections in humans.
- **Phase 2:** The disease has caused proven infection in humans.
- **Phase 3:** Small clusters of disease occur in humans but do not affect entire communities.
- **Phase 4:** The disease affects entire communities. The disease now qualifies as an epidemic, but the risk for a pandemic, although increased, is not certain.
- **Phase 5:** Spread of disease between humans is occurring in more than one country in a region. The Ebola virus outbreak of 2014 is an example of this phase; cases affected communities in several different west African countries.

- **Phase 6:** Community-level outbreaks are in at least one additional country in a different region. In the case of Ebola, cases in North America and Europe didn't originate there and the infection didn't take hold locally in any significant manner. Therefore, Ebola failed to meet the criteria for a pandemic. Influenza, however, commonly reaches pandemic status on an annual basis.

MAJOR PANDEMICS: A SHORT HISTORY

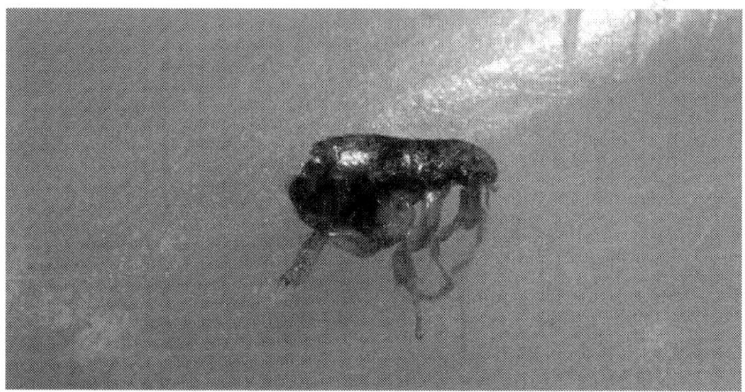

Fleas serve as vectors for the Plague

Ask people about the last pandemic and most will say it was the "Spanish Flu" of 1918-9. Certainly, that outbreak is a well-known example, but pandemics have occurred throughout history. At least three or four are identified every century. It can even be argued that we've experienced more than one just in the last few years.

Ancient Pandemics

Pandemics came with regularity (and great severity) in ancient times. Several pandemics became infamous due, not only to their deadly nature, but also their effect on Western civilization. The most prominent of these include:

The Great Plague of Athens: The plague of Athens took place between the years 430-426 BC during the onset of the Peloponnesian War. Thought to have arisen in Africa, the plague killed a third of the Athenian population and an estimated 300,000 people throughout the Mediterranean. Indeed, it is thought to have brought about the end of the Greek Golden Age. Contemporary writers reported that plague symptoms included high fever, blistered skin, bilious vomiting, intestinal ulcerations, and diarrhea. Although it is unknown what disease caused the epidemic, Typhus or Typhoid Fever are thought to be the prime candidates.

The Antonine Plague: Named for the Roman emperor and philosopher Marcus Aurelius Antoninus, the outbreak began in 165 AD and lasted 15 years. An estimated five million people died from what is now thought to have been smallpox. It's believed to have begun in Mesopotamia (modern-day Iraq) and spread all the way to Rome by soldiers returning from campaigns. At one point during the pandemic, an estimated 2,000 Romans died each day. The emperor himself is thought to have been one of the victims.

The Plague of Justinian: In the year 541 AD, rats from Egyptian grain boats brought a pestilence to the Eastern Roman Empire that would ultimately leave approximately 25 million people dead. Even the emperor Justinian I, for whom the plague was named, was infected, although he survived. As many as 5,000 people died per day in the capital city of Constantinople. Before the outbreak was over, about 40 percent of the city's population was dead—so many and so quickly that bodies were left unburied in piles. The entire Mediterranean coast lost about a quarter of its population. Modern experts now believe that the outbreak was the first recorded case of the bubonic plague.

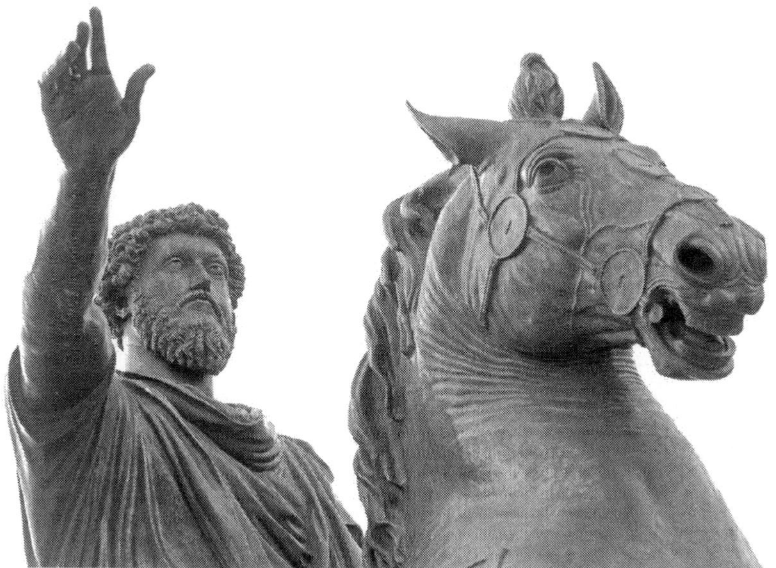

Emperor Marcus Aurelius Antoninus, pandemic victim

The Black Death: Bubonic plague came to the West via sea lanes in the 14th century. From 1347 to 1351, the disease depopulated Europe and most of the world. 75-150 million deaths are attributed to it at a time when there were about 450 million people total on the planet. Half of Europe died in a span of only four years.

The rest of the middle ages was wracked with waves of plague pandemics. Over time, it became known as the "**Black Death**" for the color of lumps (called "**buboes**") in the armpits and groins of the victims. It was so devastating that, although it's been hundreds of years since the last pandemic of the disease, most people in modern times have heard of it.

Modern Pandemics

Despite advances in identifying pathogens and medical research, pandemics still took a major toll on the world's population. Indeed, they do so even today. Some of the deadlier ones include:

Modern Plague: A major pandemic of plague began in China and Hong Kong in the 1860s. Ports around the world experienced outbreaks of the disease for the next 20 years, eventually leading to 10 million deaths.

Although the exact mechanisms of bacterial disease weren't well-known at the time, scientists were able to identify a bacterium (*Yersinia pestis*) as the infectious agent. They also rightly determined that it was transmitted by infected fleas on rats.

Although the pandemic eventually died out, infection with Yersinia pestis spread to rodent populations throughout the world. As such, plague became **endemic** to many rural areas. Even today, several cases are reported every year in the western United States.

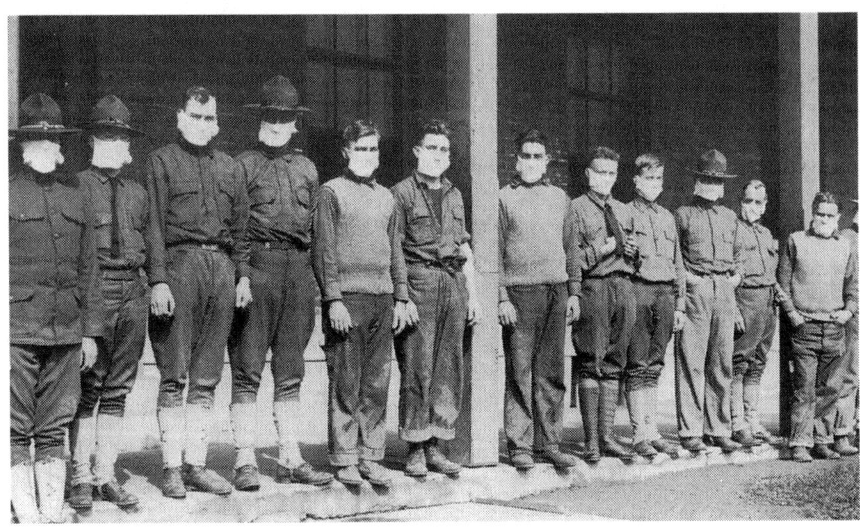

The Spanish Flu hastened the end of WWI

The Spanish Flu of 1918. As WWI was grinding to a close, a new strain of influenza began to appear simultaneously in multiple countries around the world. The disease spread quickly due to the cramped conditions that troops on both sides had to endure. Indeed, the problems it caused may have helped bring about the end of hostilities. It was called The Spanish Flu despite the fact that it didn't actually come from Spain.

The Spanish Flu made it all the way to North America but burned out quickly in late 1919 for unknown reasons. Anywhere from 3-20% of the people afflicted perished from the disease. In total, 50-100 million people are believed to have died, with perhaps 25 million of those deaths coming in the first few months of the outbreak.

HIV/AIDS: Due to a virus that attacks the immune system, Human Immunodeficiency Virus is commonly referred to as HIV. The infection led to Acquired Immune Deficiency Syndrome, also called AIDS. While medicine has made great strides in dealing with this disease in developed countries, it is still raging in many parts of Africa, where it originated. Over 30 years, at least 60 million people had been infected by AIDS and 25 million have died. In 2008 an estimated 1.2 million Americans were HIV-positive, but Sub-Saharan Africa alone was home to 22.9 million cases, with one in five adults infected. About 35.3 million people were believed to have HIV according to a study performed in 2012.

Although not reaching the level of the rogue's gallery above, there are many other diseases that have caused pandemics. Cholera, a diarrheal disease, was first seen in India and has since caused millions of cases a year and millions of deaths over time. It was especially bad in Haiti after the earthquake in that country in 2010. Measles, tuberculosis, typhus, and even syphilis caused pandemics over the years.

The Next Pandemic

What disease will be the most likely candidate to cause the next pandemic? The answer depends on the level of attention that we place on prevention. The return of historically important pandemics like The Plague and Cholera are still very real possibilities, especially in areas that have limited access to modern medicine. Antibiotics that can nip infections in the bud may decrease the risk, but will they be available in large quantities?

Could the next pandemic come from a more recently identified disease? This was the question we posed when this book was first published in late 2018. The answer would come in an emphatic and deadly manner when the 2020 pandemic emerged. When we reported on the new virus, it had not yet been named and only 60 cases were reported in China without a single fatality. By late 2021, hundreds of millions were infected and several million died from the disease.

We correctly predicted that the next pandemic would be viral. Other candidates had come and gone in the early 21st century. Ebola was a major epidemic, but can the organism that causes it live outside certain climates? Sudden Acute Respiratory Syndrome, also known as SARS, was an issue in the East some years ago and is a reason why you see images of many Asians wearing face masks in public. Middle East Respiratory Syndrome, or MERS, is a lethal disease related to SARS that is a problem in many middle eastern countries that employ foreign workers.

A virus called Chikungunya is carried by mosquitoes and has ranged far and wide over the Caribbean and other tropical regions in the recent past. Chikungunya causes fever as well as stomach and joint problems. Recovery sometimes takes months but, fortunately, the disease doesn't cause many deaths.

Zika virus became the newest member of the pandemic club in 2015-6, when it traveled from French Polynesia and Asia to Brazil. Spread by mosquitoes, Zika was a relatively mild infection for most adults. Thousands of newborns, however, were identified with brain defects at birth as a result of the virus.

Despite the ravages of the 2020 pandemic, perhaps the highest risk for a pandemic disease is still Influenza. There are many different varieties and the virus mutates frequently. In 2009, the Swine Flu epidemic killed 200,000 people. Other influenza strains are being identified every year, with each having the potential to become widespread outbreaks.

HOW INFECTIONS SPREAD

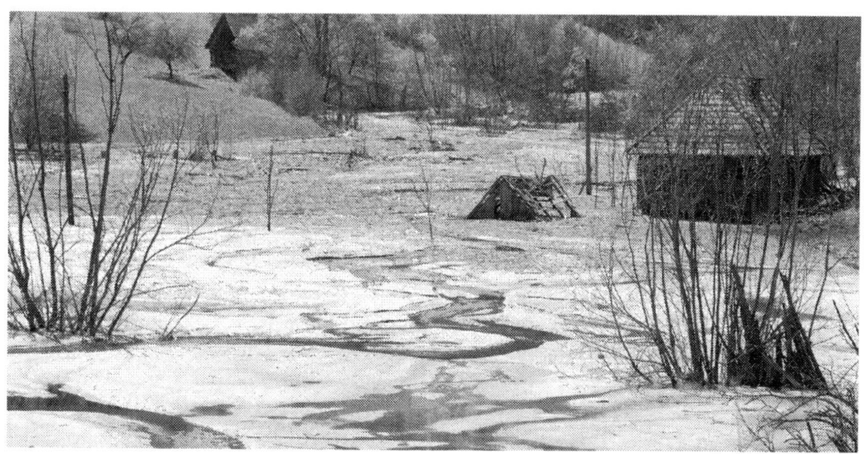

A pandemic isn't a pandemic, by definition, unless it spreads. So how are infectious diseases transmitted throughout a community? Here are the most common methods that an infection takes hold in a community:

Ingestion—Eating infected animals is a common cause for an infection to spread to humans. For example, bats and monkeys are part of the diet of many people in Africa; these animals are known carriers of the Ebola virus. Primitive safety standards led to undercooked meat spreading the disease.

Contamination of water and food is responsible for "poisoning" outbreaks that make the news every day. In 2011, millions of pounds of turkey meat contaminated with *Salmonella* were discarded after more than 100 consumers required hospitalization. In 2018 alone, tainted products ranging from lettuce to ground beef were responsible for several outbreaks.

Inhalation—Inhaling a pathogen is perhaps the most dangerous form of transmission from a sheer numbers standpoint. The infection spreads through air by breathing in droplets from the afflicted. These are formed when body fluids from sick patients become aerosolized in coughs and sneezes. Those in close contact with these people are at risk for the germ to enter through the mouth, nose, or eyes. Most epidemics of respiratory illnesses like influenza are spread this way.

Injection—From needle sticks or other medical items. Hepatitis is a disease commonly passed by injection of "recreational" drugs, but almost any blood-borne illness is a candidate. The opioid epidemic currently raging in the U.S. is causing more and more cases to be transmitted this way. Certain hospital-based infections may be inadvertently spread via injection.

Absorption—Disease can be spread by touching secretions from the infected and then your mouth, eyes, or an open sore. People, especially children, are notoriously lax when it comes to the practice of touching their face with their hands. To see how often this happens, just look at the average person and count the number of times they touch their face over, say, a half hour. The risk of infection by absorption indicates just how important it is for caregivers to wear gloves and masks.

Sexually Transmitted—An entire group of infections are well-known to be spread from the semen and other bodily secretions of infected persons during sexual activity. Syphilis is a sexually transmitted disease (**STD**). From the 1400s to the early 1900s, it was a scourge of almost every civilized country and is currently making a comeback in the United States.

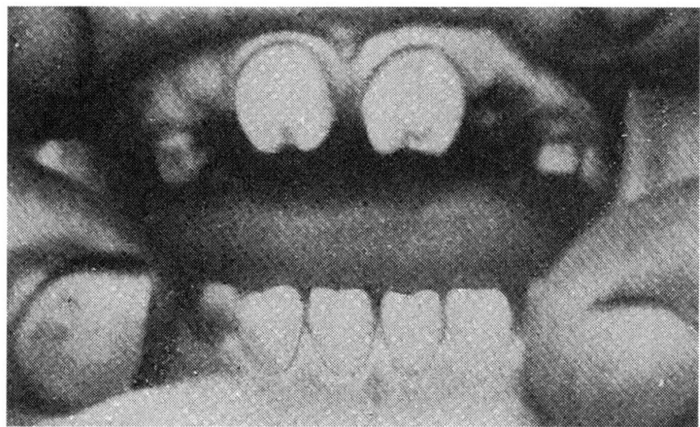

Notched teeth seen in congenital syphilis

Pregnancy-Related—Infections may be passed from mother to fetus. Gonorrhea is a common STD which, if contracted during a pregnancy, increases the risk of miscarriage or preterm delivery. A baby born while the mother has an active gonorrhea infection can develop joint infections, blindness, or worse. Other diseases passed this way include HIV, Syphilis, Zika, and Ebola. All can have dire consequences for the fetus and newborn.

Complacency—Lack of attention to infection control is probably the biggest reason for the spread of pandemic diseases. In 2014, nurses at a Texas hospital were infected when an Ebola victim traveled to the United States. Lax hospital protocols were blamed. At one point during the epidemic in West Africa, U.S. hospitals were unprepared for possible spread to North America. So unprepared, in fact, that there was a total of only 19 isolation beds that could handle a highly contagious disease in the entire country.

Due to the hard lessons learned, this issue has been corrected in the U.S. Most of the world, however, is still poorly prepared to deal with a major epidemic.

SECTION 2

BACTERIAL DISEASES

Infectious disease outbreaks caused by bacterial organisms have been a part of the human experience since before recorded history. **Cholera** is one example. A disease seen in areas with sanitation issues, it has ravaged entire communities in both the distant and recent past. Although the grand majority of bacteria are harmless, numerous bacterial species exist that can be life-threatening to humans.

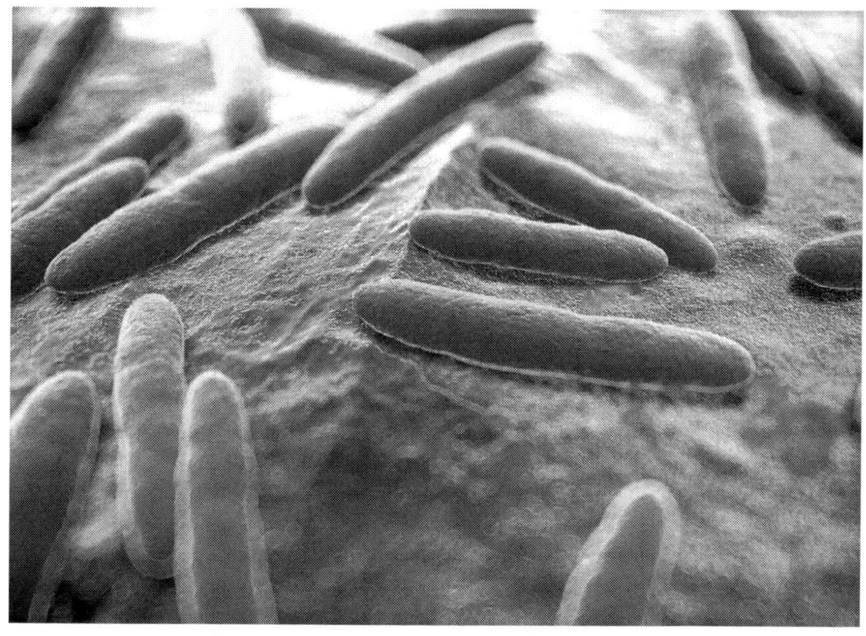

COMMON BACTERIAL DISEASES

Thanks to medical advancements like antibiotics, some pathogens were more dangerous in the past than they are now. Underdeveloped countries and areas recovering from disasters continue, however, to be plagued by bacterial disease.

Below are some bacterial and protozoal diseases, each with a description of symptoms and possible treatments. They are separated into those that are common now in developed countries or *will* be if a modern society is thrown off the power grid due to some catastrophe.

Of course, some diseases in the "will be" group are running rampant right now in nations with weak medical infrastructures. Although they may not be major issues in the United States, millions of cases are reported in areas of Africa and Asia.

The infections listed aren't the only diseases that you should know about; together, however, they represent hundreds of millions of cases a year worldwide. It should be noted that, although antibiotics are mentioned in the descriptions below, they and their alternatives will be discussed individually in more detail later in this book.

EAR, EYE, NOSE, AND THROAT

Eye Infections

The most common eye infection is called "**conjunctivitis**." The conjunctiva is the thin membrane that covers the white of your eye. Conjunctivitis is an inflammation which causes the affected eye to become red, itchy, and tearful. Although conjunctivitis, also called "Pink Eye," can be caused by chemical irritation or a foreign body, viruses and bacteria are also possibilities.

Conjunctivitis caused by a microbe is more likely to produce a milky white discharge.

Bacteria that may cause pink eye include *Staphylococcus aureus*, *Streptococcus pneumoniae*, and *Haemophilus influenzae*. Occasionally, organisms that are usually associated with sexual transmission, like *Chlamydia trachomatis* and *Neisseria gonorrhoeae*, may be to blame.

Once you have identified what you believe to be a bacterial conjunctivitis, it is important to prevent its spread as it is extremely contagious, especially among children. Strict attention to frequent hand washing is the most effective method of keeping the infection under control.

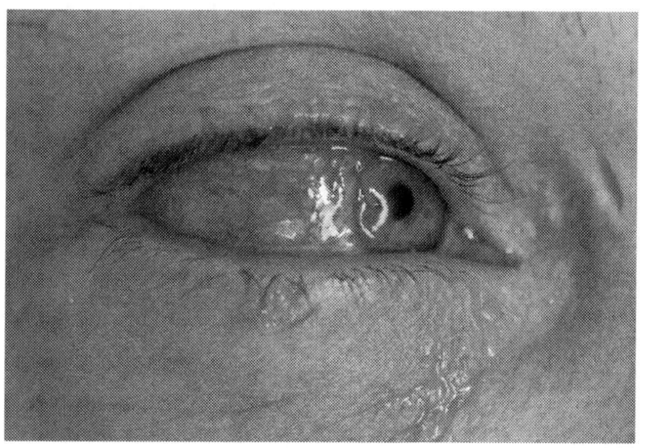

Bacterial conjunctivitis

Medication for eye infections usually comes in the form of eye drops with antibiotics like tobramycin. Always ask your eye doctor for samples if available. When using eye drops, be sure to keep the bottle two or three inches above you eye to avoid contamination.

Oral antibiotics are rarely used for this condition in normal times, but Doxycycline 100mg twice a day for a week or less should effectively relieve bacterial conjunctivitis. Warm moist compresses often improve the discomfort associated with the infection.

Another common infection of the eye is known as a "**stye**." A stye presents as a bump on the eyelid most closely resembling a pimple. It may be on the outside or inside near the eyelashes or tear duct. The area will appear red, swollen, warm, and uncomfortable. Some notice a crusty discharge, especially upon awakening.

Styes are caused by a blocked gland near an eyelash due to an accumulation of the bacteria *Staphylococcus aureus*. Luckily, styes do not affect vision unless they become very large, which is a rarity. Normally, they tend to grow, "pop" and drain, and go away after a few days. Despite this, there is often a sense of urgency to deal with it, due to discomfort and cosmetic appearance.

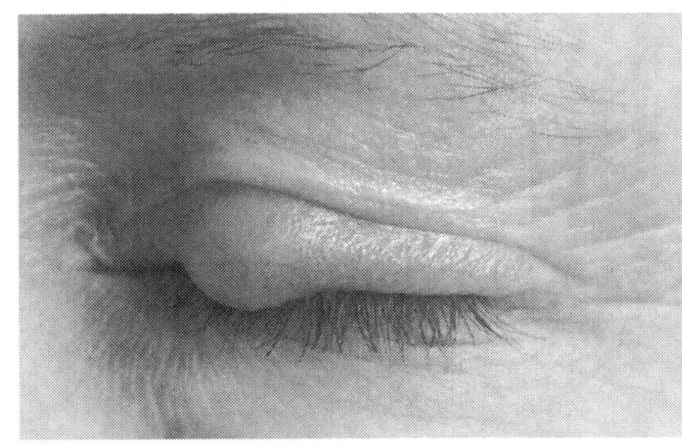

Stye

A stye is sometimes confused with a condition called a "**chalazion**" that is unrelated to infection. A chalazion is caused by the blockage of eyelid gland ducts. Normally, these glands, located in the center of the inside of the eyelid, excrete an oily substance that lubricates the eye.

Styes develop quickly, but a chalazion forms over a longer time (sometimes in the area of a previous stye). Unlike styes, a chalazion is painless, but just as disfiguring. Like styes, they tend to resolve on their own, although it may take months.

The simplest way to deal with a stye is to apply warm moist compresses for 10 minutes twice or three times a day. This strategy helps the stye drain faster. In between, clean gently with a warm moist cotton swab. Antibiotic eye solutions used for conjunctivitis will help to speed recovery. For prevention, perform eyelid scrubs regularly with a warm moist cotton ball and a small amount of baby shampoo.

If a stye spreads to the rest of the face, it becomes what is called "**cellulitis**." In this circumstance, oral antibiotics in the penicillin, cephalosporin, or macrolide families (discussed later in this book) are appropriate.

Ear Infections

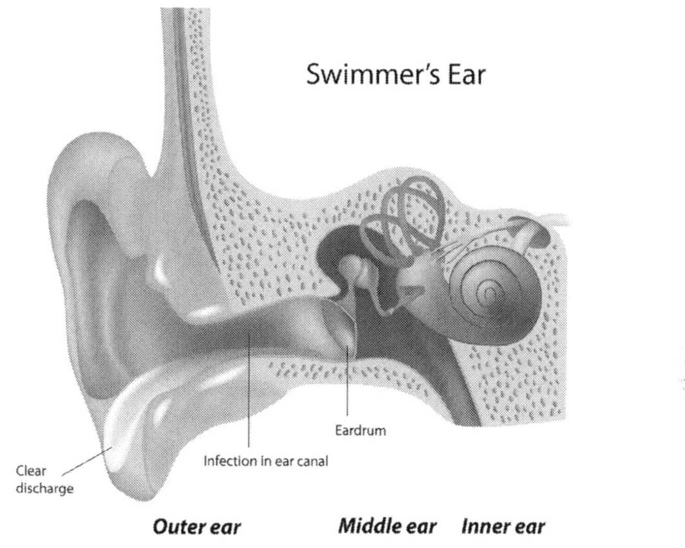

Ear Anatomy with Otitis Externa

Ear infections (also called "**otitis**") more often affect children than adults. The ear is divided into outer, middle, and inner areas, each of which may become infected. Close attention to signs and symptoms may help diagnose the location. The majority are caused by either *streptococcus pneumoniae* or *haemophilus influenza*.

Otitis Externa: Also known as "Swimmer's Ear," otitis externa is an infection of the outer ear canal, and most commonly affects children aged 4 -14 years old. Cases peak during summer months, when most people go swimming. Bacteria accumulate in the ear canal and multiply in water or sweat.

Symptoms of otitis externa include earache, itching, redness, drainage, and a "full sensation" in the ear canal. Some notice ringing (also called "tinnitus"). In some cases, hearing may be impaired. One clue that you're dealing with otitis externa is that earache pain is worsened by pulling on the ear itself.

Swimmer's ear is treated by cleaning out the ear canal with a solution of acetic acid (vinegar), which changes the pH and helps kill the bacteria. Afterwards, Polysporin antibiotic ear drops with lidocaine (for pain relief) may be effective. Oral antibiotics are thought to be less effective than ear drops for external ear infections.

Otitis Media: The most common cause of earache is an infection of the middle ear, called "otitis media." It is prevalent among infants and toddlers who breastfeed while lying flat. Symptoms include:

- Earache made worse when lying down.
- Fever
- Loss of balance
- Drainage of fluid
- Decreased hearing
- Loss of balance
- Crying, irritability, difficulty sleeping in infants and toddlers

One clue, especially with young children, is that they constantly hold or pull on the affected ear.

A useful medical tool for the medic in the diagnosis of ear conditions is the otoscope. It allows you to see the inside of the ear canal up to and including the outer surface of the eardrum.

Normally, the eardrum is shiny and grayish. When there is an infection in the middle ear canal, the eardrum will appear dull due to pus or inflammatory pressing against the inside.

Treatment may include oral antibiotics such as Amoxicillin and pain meds like ibuprofen. Antibiotic ear drops are also available. In order to get the most effect from the medicine, place the drops with the patient lying on the side opposite to the affected ear. They should stay in that position for 5 minutes to completely coat the ear canal.

Otitis Interna: Inner ear canal infections are often characterized by dizziness, also known as "**vertigo**." Patients with otitis interna commonly feel nauseous as well as dizzy. Treatment with diazepam (Valium), meclizine (Antivert) or Dimenhydrinate (Dramamine) can help with symptoms. Amoxicillin is commonly used as antibiotic therapy.

Bacterial Sinusitis

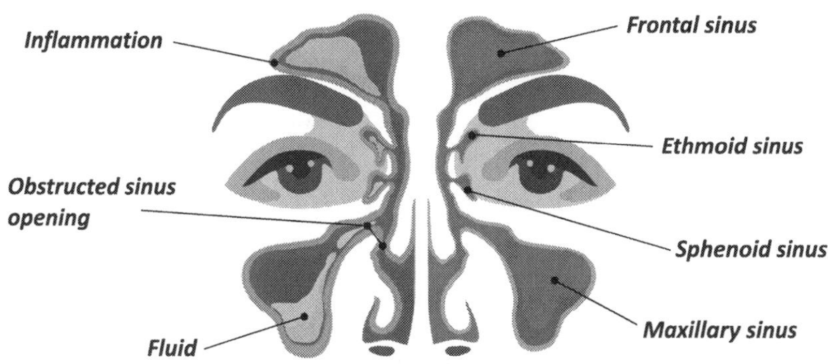

Facial Sinuses

Sinuses are spaces in the bones of the face or skull that connect to the nasal cavities. Sinus infections (also called "sinusitis") can occur as a result of a virus or bacteria. When bacterial in origin, the organisms involved are often *streptococcus pneumoniae* or *haemophilus influenzae.*

Symptoms depend on the particular sinus affected, but may include some of the following:

- Facial pressure or pain (often one-sided)
- Nasal congestion
- Fever
- Nasal drainage

- Cough
- Fatigue
- Upper dental pain
- Ear fullness/pressure
- Fatigue

Although the above symptoms may occur regardless of whether the pathogen is viral or bacterial, consider bacteria if symptoms are persistent or worsen after an initial improvement.

Treatment consists of nasal decongestants like pseudoephedrine, phenylephrine, and oxymetazoline hydrochloride. Be aware of excessive use of decongestants as some become dependent on them. Antibiotic treatment is usually Amoxicillin, Clarithromycin, or Azithromycin for 14 days.

Strep Throat/Tonsillitis

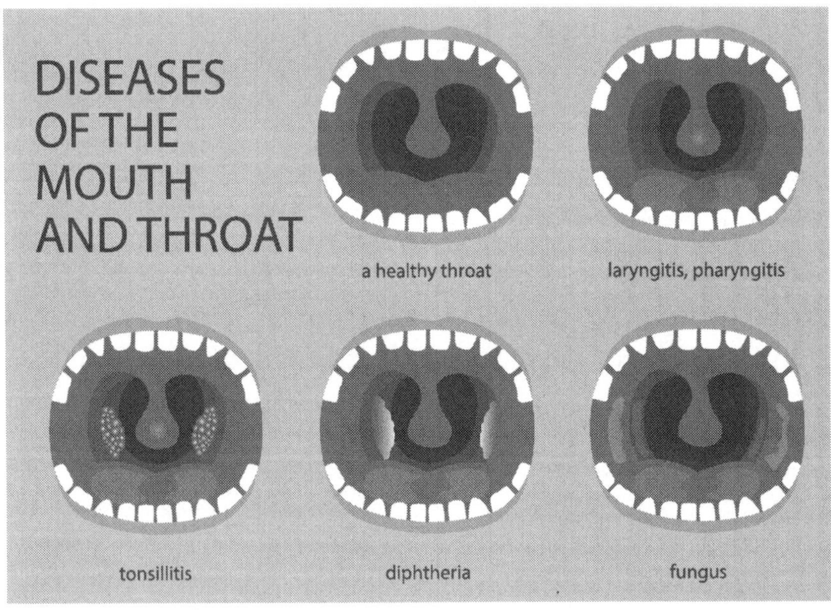

There are two types of *streptococcus*, "group A" and "group B." Group A *Streptococcus pyogenes* causes a number of different types of infections, including "strep throat." Strep throat is a form of sore throat (also called "**pharyngitis**") which inflames the tonsils. You will see white spots on them or the back of the throat. Other symptoms include are a high fever, redness, and, of course, a sore throat.

Group A strep is responsible for a number of other infections:

- **Scarlet fever**—a sickness that causes a bright red rash and fever (hence the name) and often follows a strep throat infection.
- **Impetigo**—a common skin infection characterized by red sores that burst, ooze yellow fluid, and then crust over.
- **Cellulitis**—a skin and soft tissue infection that causes redness, pain, local warmth, and swelling.
- Some cases of **necrotizing fasciitis**—an extreme form of cellulitis that destroys tissue and may lead to amputation.

Group B strep can cause serious issues as well, such as blood infections, pneumonia, urinary infections, and meningitis. It is especially dangerous in newborns.

A number of antibiotics can be used to treat mild-moderate cases of the above, including penicillins, cephalosporins, lincosamides, and other families of drugs. Intravenous antibiotics and surgical intervention may be required for severe infections like necrotizing fasciitis.

RESPIRATORY

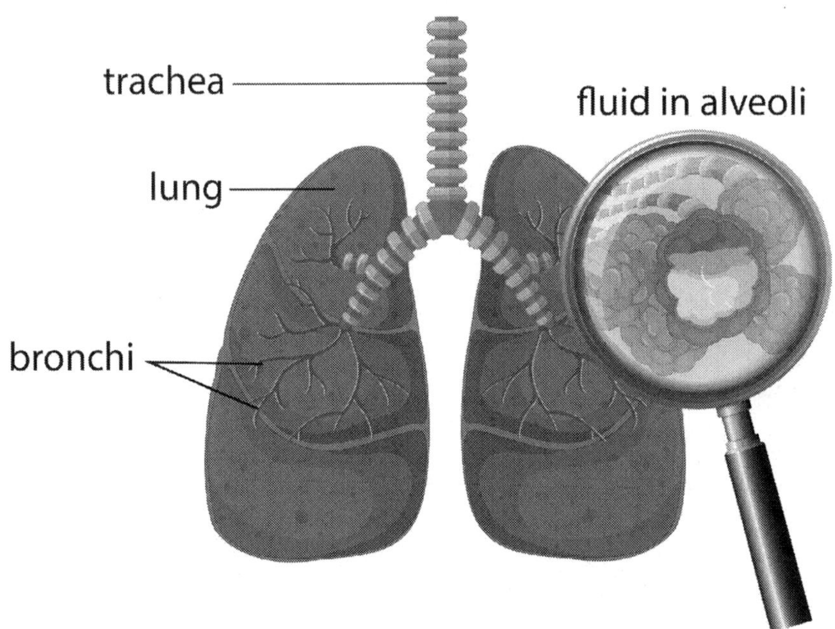

Pneumonia with fluid accumulation in alveoli

Bronchitis And Pneumonia

It's important to realize that the majority of respiratory infections, including the flu and the common cold, are caused by viruses and do not improve with the use of antibiotics. Some infections of the respiratory tract are bacterial in origin, however; others are **secondary infections** that invade a weakened victim of a viral illness. These tend to be in the lower airways (called "**bronchitis**") or in the lung tissue itself (called "**pneumonia**"). Bacterial pneumonia has been given the dubious title "the old man's friend" because it stops the suffering of the elderly (by ending their lives).

There are many different microbes that cause pneumonia and bronchitis. The **incubation period** for most lower respiratory infections is only one to three days. This means that you will begin to experience ill effects from the disease very soon after you are first exposed.

Whether bacterial or viral in origin, fever is a common symptom of respiratory infections. Temperatures tend to be higher and get worse over time when bacteria are the cause. With a viral infection, fevers usually improve after a few days. A period of improvement followed by the return of a high fever may signal a **secondary infection** with bacteria.

The lungs have small air sacs called "**alveoli**" that absorb oxygen from inhaled air. In pneumonia, alveoli become filled with inflammatory fluid, making it difficult to transport oxygen to body tissues. Symptoms classically seen include cough, fever, phlegm, shortness of breath, and chest pain.

Bronchitis happens when the airways that carry oxygen from your windpipe to your lungs become inflamed. The lining becomes clogged with mucus, causing cough, wheezes, and phlegm which may be yellow or greyish.

Although a number of respiratory infections may be associated with a certain color of mucus, it is not always a sure diagnosis. Yellow **sputum**, for example, has been associated with bronchitis, but the phlegm is just as likely to be whitish or grey in color. Yellow sputum may also be a sign of pneumonia or even non-infectious conditions like asthma.

Many different bacteria have been implicated as the pathogen in pneumonia, but a few are more common than others. It should be noted that, without lab studies, many pneumonias caused by different pathogens appear very similar. It is sometimes a challenge to choose the right therapy.

Some bacterial types of pneumonia are listed below. Besides the usual signs and symptoms, we have included some additional clues that may help make the **diagnosis**. Treatment options are included, but described in much more detail in the antibiotics section of this book.

Streptococcus pneumoniae: also called "pneumococcal pneumonia," it is usually associated with rusty-colored sputum. The most common type of bacterial pneumonia, it was treated primarily with penicillin (beta-lactam) family drugs but resistant strains may be more susceptible to sulfonamides, macrolides, or fluoroquinolones.

Legionella pneumophila: associated with abdominal pain, diarrhea, and, in the elderly, confusion. Recently found to be due to contamination of cooling units in some inner-city housing projects. A macrolide like azithromycin or erythromycin is a reasonable choice.

Klebsiella pneumoniae: associated with dark bloody sputum that is reminiscent of cherry or red currant preserves. Klebsiella is actually a normal inhabitant of the human skin and intestines; it is dangerous, however, if it invades lung tissue. Although fluoroquinolones may be effective, intravenous antibiotics are usually required.

Mycoplasma pneumoniae: associated with ear symptoms, swelling of nearby lymph nodes, and joint pain. Was once known as "walking pneumonia," since symptoms weren't severe enough to cause a patient to be bedridden. Mycoplasma species differ from other bacteria in that they lack a cell wall. Since many antibiotics like penicillin kill bacteria by targeting cell wall synthesis, mycoplasma is naturally resistant to them. A macrolide like azithromycin or erythromycin is preferable.

Haemophilus Influenzae: Presents like a cold at first with associated low-grade fevers. This descends to the lungs in a matter of days, with wheezing, difficulty breathing, and grey-beige sputum. Cough may persist for weeks unless treated. Treatment: Penicillin (beta-lactam) family drugs often used as first line, but sulfa drugs, tetracyclines, fluoroquinolones, and macrolide antibiotics are also options.

We mention individual bacterial species and their signs because different antibiotics are used based on the type. In austere settings without access to modern medicine, you'll be making an educated guess as to what bacteria might be involved (or if it is bacterial at all). This is a hard reality in remote locations, but one that must be faced with determination.

Azithromycin, Cephalexin, and Sulfa drugs may be acceptable in scenarios where no lab identification is possible. Resistance to amoxicillin and some other penicillin family drugs has led to their becoming less useful, at least in the United States. Intravenous medications are almost always needed for severe cases.

Epiglottitis

The epiglottis is a structure at the base of your tongue. It works as a valve to prevent food from going down your windpipe as you eat and drink. When the epiglottis becomes infected, it can swell and block your airways. Although this condition is more common in children, it is increasingly being seen in adults and represents an emergency in both groups. Adult cases seem to develop more slowly than pediatric ones.

Epiglottitis can start showing symptoms as soon as one to three days after exposure to the bacteria. The symptoms of epiglottitis seen commonly include:

- High fever
- Sore throat
- Difficulty breathing
- Hoarseness
- Agitation

Some report a lessening of symptoms when upright or leaning forward. This condition has been associated with **croup**, also called "**laryngotracheobronchitis**"; croup, however, is usually caused by a virus. Staph, Strep, and Hemophilus may be involved in rare bacterial cases.

Epiglottitis is treated by third-generation cephalosporins like Ceftriaxone intravenously. In austere settings where modern IV therapy is not an option, amoxicillin/clavulanic acid or clindamycin may be considered, although swallowing difficulties may make this strategy problematic.

Whooping Cough

Whooping Cough, also called "**Pertussis,**" is an infection of the airways caused by the bacteria *Bordetella pertussis*. The microbe attaches to the lining of the upper respiratory system and releases toxins which cause swelling. More and more cases of this illness are being reported in certain parts of the United States.

After an average of 7-10 days (range 4-42 days) of incubation, pertussis begins as a cold or flu-like syndrome with nasal congestion, low-grade fever, and mild cough. In infants, a pause between breaths (called "**apnea**") may become noticeable.

After one or two weeks of the above, full blown pertussis becomes apparent. You will see violent coughing fits (known as "**paroxysms**"). These occur fast and furious until all the air in the lungs is expended. A forceful inhalation then occurs, causing a high-pitched "whoop" sound. Many patients vomit. So much coughing occurs that pertussis sufferers end up totally exhausted.

Resolution of the infection is slow and total recovery may take 10 weeks or more. In China, pertussis is known as the "100-day cough." Adults and teenagers seem to have a milder disease course than young children.

It should be noted that whooping cough is highly contagious, passing from person to person in air droplets from the sheer number of coughing fits. Infected people should be isolated for at least two weeks after the cough begins. Antibiotics like azithromycin, erythromycin, and sulfamethoxazole-trimethoprim (sulfa) may shorten the amount of time someone is contagious.

ABDOMINAL

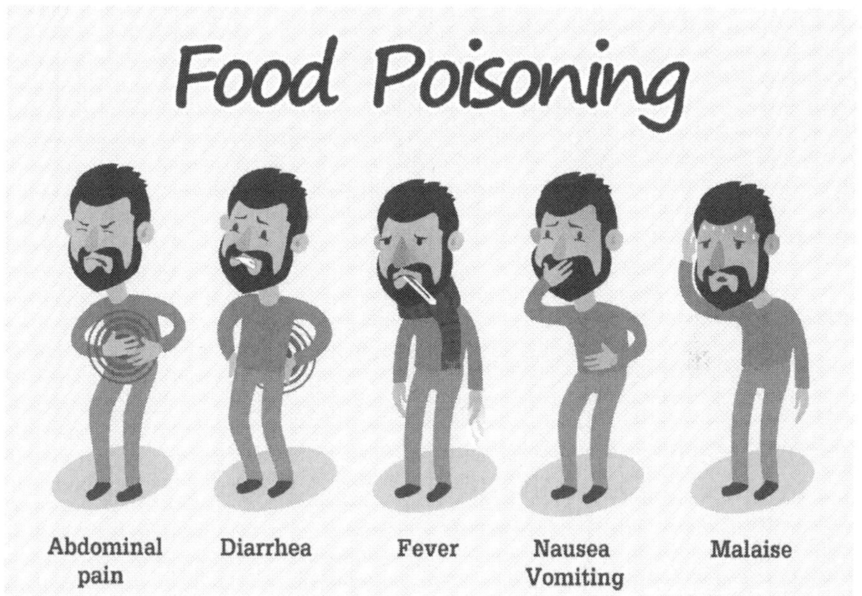

Traveler's Diarrhea

An inflammation of the small intestine most commonly caused by the Bacterium Escherichia coli, commonly known as "E. coli." Most strains of this bacteria are normal inhabitants of the human intestinal tract, but one (E. coli O157:H7) produces a toxin (the "**Shiga**" toxin) that can cause severe food poisoning. Shiga is so toxic that it has been classified as a bioterror agent.

Sudden onset of watery diarrhea, often with blood, develops within one to three days of exposure accompanied by fever, gas, and abdominal cramping. Rapid rehydration and treatment with antibiotics such as Azithromycin, Sulfa drugs, and Ciprofloxacin is helpful. It should be noted that the CDC (Centers for Disease Control and Prevention) no longer recommends taking antibiotics in advance of a journey. It does, however, suggest that Pepto-Bismol (Bismuth Subsalicylate), two tablets four times a day, may help in prevention.

Campylobacter Food Poisoning

The second most common cause of foodborne illness in the U.S. after *Salmonella*, *Campylobacter jejuni* resides in the intestinal tract of chickens. The bacteria cause sickness when meat is undercooked or improperly processed. Infection is characterized by bloody diarrhea, fever, nausea, and cramping which begins two to five days after exposure. Although it is questionable in terms of its effectiveness, Erythromycin may decrease the duration of illness if taken early.

Listeria Food Poisoning

Another form of food poisoning is caused by the bacterium *Listeria monocytogenes*. The infection is most likely to sicken the elderly and immune-deficient, as well as pregnant women and newborns.

Listeria can cause fever and diarrhea similar to other foodborne germs. When Listeria spreads beyond the intestinal tract, it is usually in pregnant women and can lead to complications like miscarriage, preterm delivery, or stillbirth. The newborn may also develop the infection, which could become life-threatening.

Various antibiotics can be used to treat listeria infection, including ampicillin, sulfa drugs, erythromycin, tetracycline, and gentamycin.

Cryptosporidiosis (Crypto)

The protozoan *Cryptosporidium* is an especially hardy organism responsible for the grand majority of those made ill by contaminated water, especially in recreational areas. Also known as "Crypto," the organism spreads when someone who is sick with the parasite goes swimming and releases a bowel movement into the water.

The incubation period averages 5-10 days after swallowing contaminated water. Those infected can become sick for weeks with watery diarrhea, stomach cramps, and vomiting. Severe or long-standing cases can damage the liver, leading to yellowing of the skin known as "**jaundice**." A respiratory version also exists where nasal congestion, hoarseness, cough, fever, and shortness of breath occur.

Crypto infections occur even in properly chlorinated pools: Chlorine takes *days* to eliminate the microbe, as compared to minutes for organisms like *E. coli* and others. Boiling works very quickly, however, to eliminate the organism. Treatment options include nitazoxanide, azithromycin and anti-diarrheal meds like loperamide (Imodium). As with any disease that may cause dehydration, fluids are important.

Giardiasis

Although not a bacterium, the protozoan *Giardia lamblia* deserves mention as the most common disease-causing parasite in the world. Although not considered "**Traveler's Diarrhea**," any backcountry traveler may find themselves a victim by drinking contaminated water. Giardia inhabits even the clearest mountain streams in U.S. national parks.

Symptoms commonly present one to two weeks after exposure. Patients complain of foul watery or greasy diarrhea, abdominal cramping, violent ("projectile") vomiting, and gas.

Giardia lamblia exists in active and inactive forms. The active form is called a "**trophozoite**"; the inactive form is referred to as a "**cyst**." Trophozoites attach to the lining of the small intestine and cause the symptoms.

Trophozoites can't live long outside a host, however, so it is the hardier cysts that spread the infection to other people. When as little as ten cysts are ingested due to contaminated water, stomach acid turns them into trophozoites and the signs and symptoms of the illness become apparent.

A course of metronidazole is a popular antibiotic used in conjunction with oral rehydration, although some newer drugs like Tinidazole have recently entered the marketplace that might be effective with just a single dose. The formula for making oral rehydration solution at home is discussed later in this book.

Appendicitis

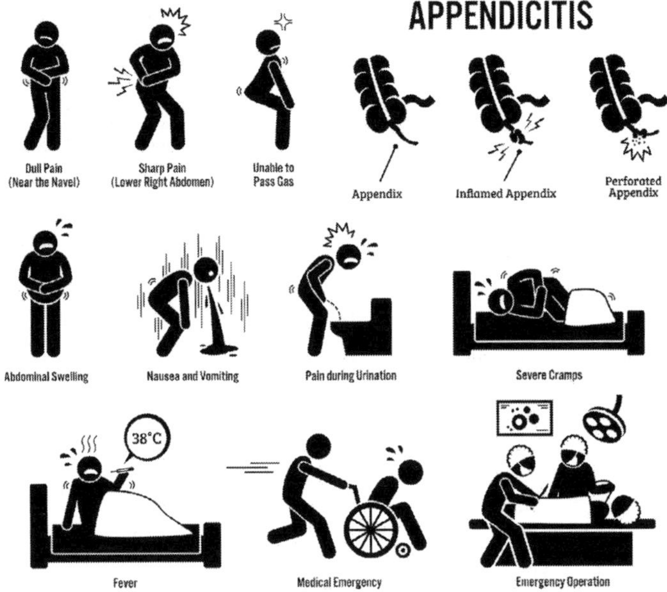

The appendix is a tubular worm-shaped piece of tissue two to four inches long. It opens into the intestine at the lower right side of the abdomen. The hollow part of the appendix may become blocked by bits of hard excrement, causing appendicitis. The suffix "itis" simply means "inflammation of"; therefore, appendicitis is "inflammation of the appendix."

An inflamed appendix is normally treated with surgical removal and, indeed, 300,000 appendectomies are performed in the United States every year. Some, however, are now suggesting antibiotic therapy for cases found early. This option would be especially useful in disaster settings where modern hospital care does not exist.

Although appendicitis is not caused by infection, an inflamed appendix can cause a life-threatening one, especially if it bursts and spills intestinal contents throughout the abdomen. This condition is known as "**peritonitis**," an inflammation of the lining of the abdominal cavity.

Appendicitis first presents with vague discomfort in the area of the belly button, also called the "**umbilicus**," but moves down to the lower right quadrant of the abdomen after 12-24 hours. The painful area on the lower right is called "**McBurney's Point**." You can find it about two thirds of the way down from the belly button to the top of the right pelvic bone. The discomfort can be so great that the patient may be reluctant to move. In addition, you will see nausea and vomiting, loss of appetite, fever and chills, and a swollen abdomen.

Treating appendicitis with antibiotics is risky, but one study showed that the majority of early appendicitis cases were able to avoid surgery. Intravenous antibiotics, such as Cefoxitin, are more effective than related oral antibiotics, such as Cephalexin. Metronidazole may be used if allergic to penicillin.

Urinary Tract Infections

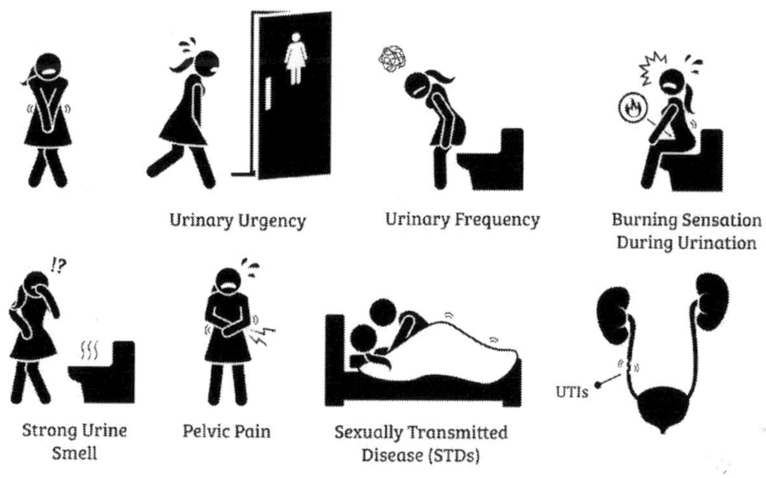

The urinary tract includes the kidneys, ureters, bladder, and urethra. You might find it interesting to know that urine is not sterile, as was once thought. Small amounts of bacteria are present in people who are asymptomatic (without symptoms).

An infection of the bladder, also known as "**cystitis**," usually affects the urethra (the tube from the bladder to the outside) as well. Although men are not immune to urinary tract infection, they are much less susceptible to them than women. One reason may be due to the length of the male urethra compared to female.

Various different organisms cause urinary tract infections: E. coli is the most common. Frequent urination, urges to go, and a stream of urine that's slow to start are classic symptoms. This triad is known as "**frequency, urgency, and hesitancy**."

Some bacteria that cause urethral inflammation, such as gonorrhea, are sexually transmitted. In men, painful urination (also called "**dysuria**") is the main symptom. Women more commonly experience discharge or lower abdominal discomfort.

If not treated, a bladder infection may ascend to the kidneys, causing an infection known as "**pyelonephritis**." Kidney infections present with different symptoms than bladder infections. Tap both sides of the back below the lowest rib with a closed fist. If a kidney is inflamed, it will cause the patient to flinch on the affected side. Fever is also more common with upper urinary tract infections.

Antibiotics useful for treating urinary tract infections include Sulfa drugs, Amoxicillin, Ciprofloxacin, and Nitrofurantoin. A non-antibiotic that works to decrease pain with urination is phenazopyridine. Although it is available without a prescription, be aware that it has the (harmless) effect of coloring the urine red or orange.

SEXUALLY TRANSMITTED

Syphilis

Syphilis is caused by the **spirochete** bacterium *Treponema pallidum*. It is the most severe bacterial infection that can be transmitted sexually and was a world-wide epidemic in centuries past.

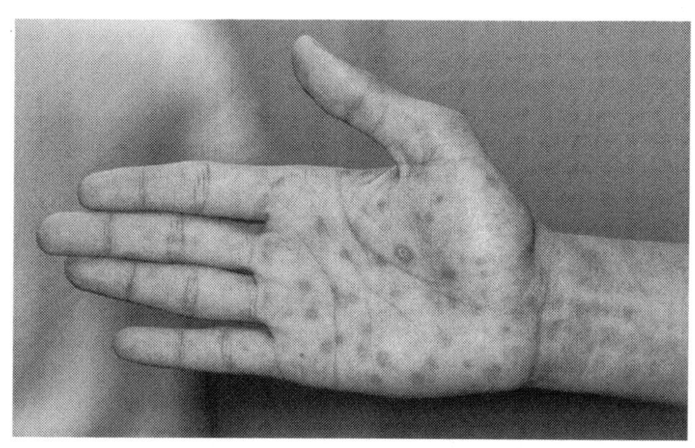

Syphilis is thought by some to be an unintentional byproduct of the discovery of the New World in 1492 by Christopher Columbus. Cases were not identified in Europe until 1494-5, when it was first described in French troops on campaign. Smallpox is an example of an epidemic disease going the other direction; it was brought by Europeans to the Americas and resulted in the decimation of Native American populations.

Syphilis develops in stages. The primary stage begins 10-90 days after exposure and manifests as a painless skin ulcer or ulcers on or near body sites commonly involved in sexual activity. This is known as a "**chancre**" and eventually goes away spontaneously after about 4-8 weeks.

The secondary stage may occur much later and appears as a red or brown rash, especially on the palms and soles. Other symptoms may include fever, sore throat, hair loss, swollen lymph nodes, and fatigue. This, too, often resolves on its own, but can lead later to tertiary syphilis. Although no longer contagious, organs begin to fail and blindness, dementia, and other dysfunctions of the nervous system occur.

When a pregnant woman is infected with syphilis, it can mean major consequences for her fetus. **Congenital** syphilis is a cause of:

- Miscarriage
- Stillbirth
- Prematurity
- Low birth weight
- Death shortly after birth

The **CDC** reports that up to 40% of babies born to women with untreated syphilis may be stillborn, or die from the infection as a newborn. A baby may be born with an enlarged liver or spleen, a low blood count (called "**anemia**"), deformed bones and teeth, blindness, deafness, or other defects.

Early diagnosis and treatment are important to avoid long-term complications from syphilis infection. Penicillin remains a popular antibiotic to cure this disease, although others have been used with success.

Gonorrhea

Another sexually transmitted disease, gonorrhea, is caused by *Neisseria gonorrhoeae*. The World Health Organization reports 88 million cases of gonorrhea a year worldwide. In the United States, it is the second most-common sexually transmitted disease. Untreated, gonorrhea may lead to damage not only of pelvic organs, but also joints, heart, and nervous system.

Although gonorrhea may be asymptomatic in some men, others experience significant burning with urination and a cloudy yellowish discharge from the penis. This usually occurs within 2-14 days after exposure. Women are less likely than men to have symptoms, although some report vaginal discharge, lower abdominal pain, and pain with intercourse. Oftentimes, the symptoms are mistaken for a bladder infection. Some cases involve symptoms relating to the throat.

Neisseria gonorrhea has proven to develop resistance to many antibiotics. Azithromycin, doxycycline, and injectable Ceftriaxone are most often used in an effort to cure the illness.

Chlamydia

Chlamydia is a bacterial infection caused by *Chlamydia trachomatis*. It is the most common sexually transmitted disease in the United States. This is likely due to the lack of early symptoms, which leads to many cases being missed by medical professionals. When symptoms do occur, they present one to three weeks after exposure and are very similar to those seen in gonorrhea.

If untreated, either chlamydia or gonorrhea can cause "pelvic inflammatory disease" which damages pelvic organs, especially in females. In males, an infection called "epididymitis" affects the male genital tract. Antibiotics options include azithromycin and doxycycline, as well as amoxicillin for patients that are pregnant.

Bacterial/Protozoan Vaginal Infections

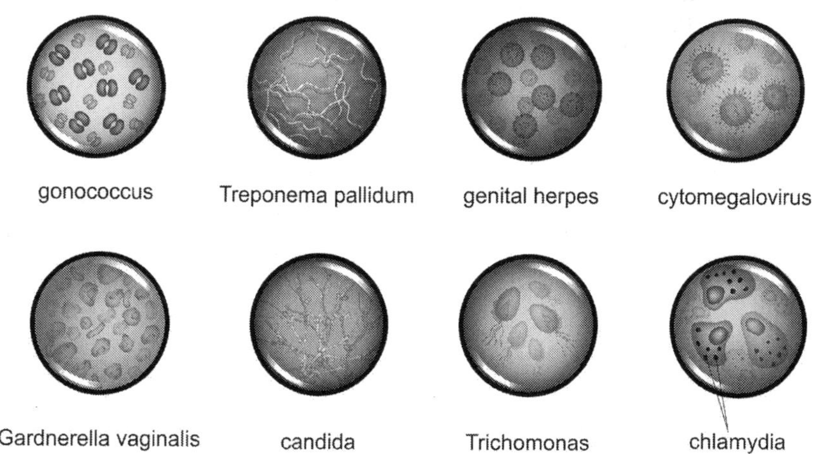

Many vaginal infections are related to fungal infections like *Candida albicans*. Others, however, are related to bacteria or protozoans that are sensitive to antibiotic therapy. These are caused by an imbalance between **normal flora** like lactobacilli and pathogens like *Gardnerella* or *Trichomonas*.

Bacterial Vaginosis (BV): According to the CDC, bacterial vaginosis is the most common vaginal infection in women ages 15-44. It is caused by Gardnerella species bacteria and shows the following symptoms in about 50% of cases:

- Watery white or gray discharge
- Vaginal itching and burning, sometimes with urination
- A "fishy" odor, often noticed during or after sex

BV can be distinguished from yeast infections by the watery nature of the discharge; Candida tends to mimic the color and consistency of cottage cheese.

Doctors commonly treat bacterial vaginosis in non-pregnant women with metronidazole or clindamycin. Either can be taken by mouth or applied as a vaginal cream or gel.

Studies show that five to seven days treatment with oral or gel metronidazole or clindamycin cream are effective treatments. As bacterial vaginosis may be associated with premature births, pregnant women can and should be given the therapy. It is thought that eating foods like yogurt that contain lactobacilli may re-establish a normal intravaginal environment.

Trichomoniasis (Trich):

Trichomoniasis is caused by an infection with a protozoan known as *Trichomonas vaginalis*. It is passed through sexual transmission. For unknown reasons, about 70% of infections are **asymptomatic**, but males and females may both experience the following about 5-28 days after exposure:

- Genital itching, redness, or irritation
- Burning with or after urination
- Discomfort during or after sex
- Penile or vaginal discharge (often yellowish or greenish)
- A "fishy" odor

Without treatment, the infection can last for months or even years. Like bacterial vaginosis, trich may cause premature labor. Metronidazole is considered the most effective antibiotic for this condition.

Bartholin's abscess

There is a pea-sized gland on each side of the vagina known as a "Bartholin's gland." They provide lubrication to the vaginal mucosa. When a Bartholin's gland becomes blocked, a cyst forms which can cause discomfort due to pressure.

When the cyst becomes infected (usually with *E. coli* or the pathogens that cause chlamydia or gonorrhea), a painful collection of pus called a "Bartholin's abscess" forms.

Warm moist compresses may allow a Bartholin's cyst or abscess to drain if used early. Once significant pain and swelling occur, an incision and drainage (discussed later under "abscess formation") may be required. For cases that recur, the walls of the cyst are sometimes stitched open to prevent re-accumulation of pus or fluid. This is known as a "marsupialization" and involves packing the open area with gauze dipped in tincture of iodine. Alternatively, placement of a tube known as a "catheter" may allow drainage during the healing process.

Antibiotics may not be necessary if the procedure is successful. When used, appropriate options include Azithromycin or doxycycline.

SKIN AND SOFT TISSUE

MRSA

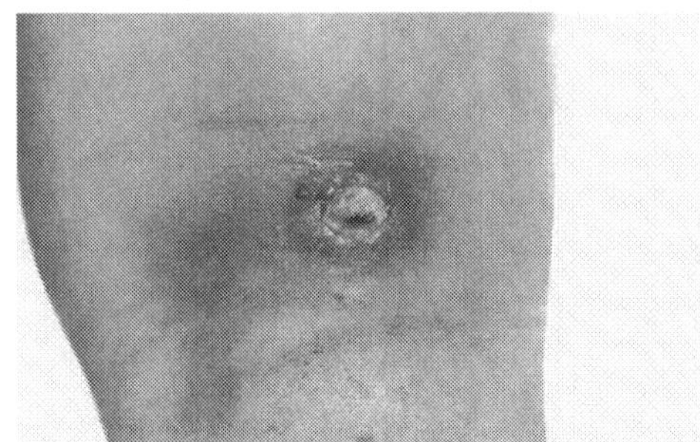

MRSA skin infection

Staphylococcus aureus is a common bacterium which can cause skin infections if it invades a cut or hair follicle. MRSA is a variant and stands for *methicillin-resistant* Staphylococcus aureus. Beside skin issues, MRSA can also cause pneumonias, infection of heart valves, soft tissue destruction, and, occasionally, an overall body infection, also known as a "**systemic**" infection.

Regular Staph aureus is so common that it inhabits the nasal cavities of 1 in 3 people. In contrast, only 2 in 100 people are thought to carry MRSA. The difference between the two is MRSA's ability to resist many antibiotics that kill regular staph pathogens.

MRSA is spread by skin contact with those infected. Three days after exposure, a skin infection with MRSA appears as a red, swollen bump on the skin that might be painful and warm to the touch. The bump may drain pus or yellowish fluid called "**exudate**." MRSA infections may also be associated with a fever.

MRSA cannot be differentiated from a boil, abscess or any other soft tissue infection (also called "**cellulitis**") with the naked eye. Cellulitis coupled with fever and cough, however, may be a clue that the bacteria has invaded the lungs. This is especially likely in those with weakened immune systems.

As the name suggests, methicillin-resistant Staph Aureus is unlikely to be eliminated by penicillin family drugs. Some strains seem to respond more to sulfa drugs, tetracyclines, and clindamycin. In many cases, however, strong intravenous drugs like vancomycin are needed. Recently, some cases are showing resistance even to the stronger therapies.

Hidradenitis Suppurativa

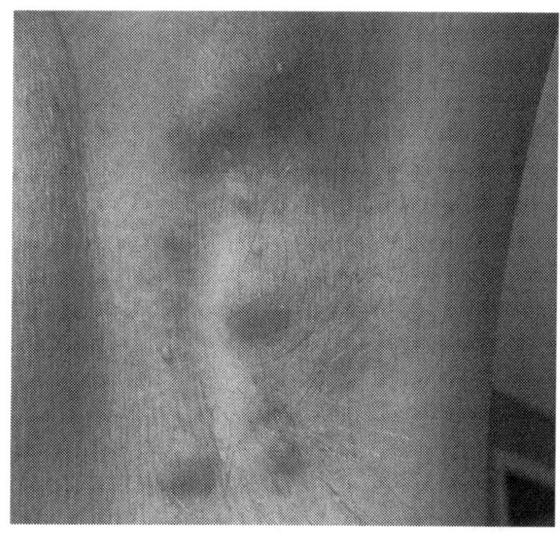

Hidradenitis suppurativa is a skin disease characterized by multiple inflamed bumps that may break open and release pus. The condition is thought to be caused by blocked sweat glands or hair follicles and not bacterial infection. The inflamed areas commonly become colonized by Staphylococcal bacteria, however.

Hidradenitis is sometimes referred to as "acne inversa" due to its appearance, but it is not actually a form of typical acne ("acne vulgaris"). Regular acne tends to involve the face, neck, and back while hidradenitis is seen most often in the underarm (also called the "axilla"), the groin, under the breasts, and between the buttocks. In addition, hidradenitis tends to be deeper and more painful.

While some people might squeeze the pimples associated with regular acne, hidradenitis suppurativa tends to spontaneously drain foul bloody pus, staining the clothing. These sometimes originate from **fistulas**, small tunnels that connect the affected gland to the skin surface.

A few popular antibiotics to treat the bacterial overgrowth in hidradenitis include tetracycline, minocycline, and clindamycin, medications also used for severe acne vulgaris. Steroids are often added to the **regimen** to decrease inflammation.

Wound Infections

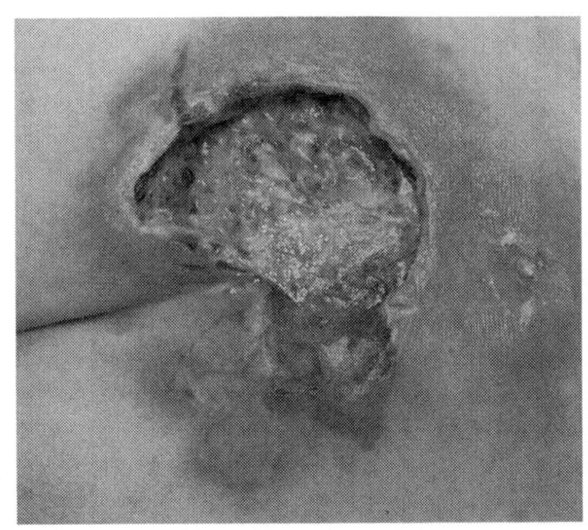

Infected bed sore

Skin is the body's armor; when it is breached, normally harmless bacteria may cause a major infection if they enter the soft tissues or circulation. The duties required for daily living in disaster settings involve physical exertion and, with it, comes the risk of injury.

Due to the availability of antibiotics, infections from minor wounds are relatively easy to treat today. Without them, even small wound infections may become life-threatening.

Infection in the soft tissues below the superficial level of the skin (the "**epidermis**") is referred to as "**cellulitis**." Below the epidermis, the main layers of soft tissue are the deep part of the skin (the "**dermis**"), the subcutaneous fat, the muscle layers, and their attendant blood vessels and nerves. Boils and abscesses are types of cellulitis characterized by a collection of pus under the skin.

The bacteria that cause cellulitis are on your skin right now. Normal flora of the surface of your skin include Staphylococcus and Group A Streptococcus. They do no harm unless the skin is broken and they invade deeper tissues. Resistant bacteria called MRSA (Methicillin-Resistant Staphylococcus Aureus) may be found on skin and cause wound infections. Other organisms that are more often associated with disease, like Pseudomonas, Vibrio, and Clostridium, may also infect soft tissues.

As an aside, **cellulitis** has nothing to do with non-infectious dimpling on the skin called "**cellulite**." The suffix "-itis" simply means "inflammation," so "cellul-itis" simply means "inflammation of the cells," appendicitis means "inflammation of the appendix," and so on...

Any injury that causes a break in the skin, including insect bites and stings, animal (or human) bites, knife or bullet wounds, surgical incisions, and more can cause cellulitis. Cellulitis can also be the result of:

- Ulcers from chronic illness, such as diabetes
- Bedsores
- Varicose veins due to poor circulation
- Intravenous drug use
- Steroid use
- Breastfeeding

The symptoms and signs of cellulitis are:

- Pain
- Redness
- Swelling
- Warmth at the site of infection
- Fever and Chills
- Drainage of pus/yellowish fluid from the area of the infection
- Foul odor

Although the body can sometimes resolve cellulitis on its own, treatment usually involves the use of antibiotics; these can be topical, oral or intravenous. Most cellulitis will improve and disappear after a 10 to 14-day course of therapy with medications in the Penicillin, Erythromycin, or Cephalosporin (Keflex) families. Amoxicillin and ampicillin are particularly popular. MRSA cellulitis can be treated with clindamycin and the sulfa drug trimethoprim-sulfamethoxazole (SMX-TMP).

If the cellulitis is in an extremity, it is helpful to keep the limb elevated. Other strategies include warm compresses or soaks to the affected area, and the use of ibuprofen (Advil) or acetaminophen (Tylenol) to decrease pain, discomfort, and fever. Regular wound cleanings twice daily are the key to full recovery. This topic is covered in more detail later in this book.

A type of cellulitis that affects new mothers is called "**mastitis**." Mastitis often occurs in the first two weeks after birth. It may often begin with a fungal infection of the skin which leads to red, sore, cracked nipples. Organisms like Staph aureus can then invade the openings in the skin or nipple ducts and cause cellulitis in underlying soft tissue. These cases present with more warmth in the area and the infection seems deeper than simple yeast infections. Fever should make you suspicious of a bacterial origin, while itching favors a fungal origin.

Treat fungal cases with clotrimazole and bacterial cellulitis with cephalexin or erythromycin. Stubborn fungal infections can be treated with fluconazole.

Abscess Formation

As mentioned previously, an **abscess** is a collection of pus under the skin.

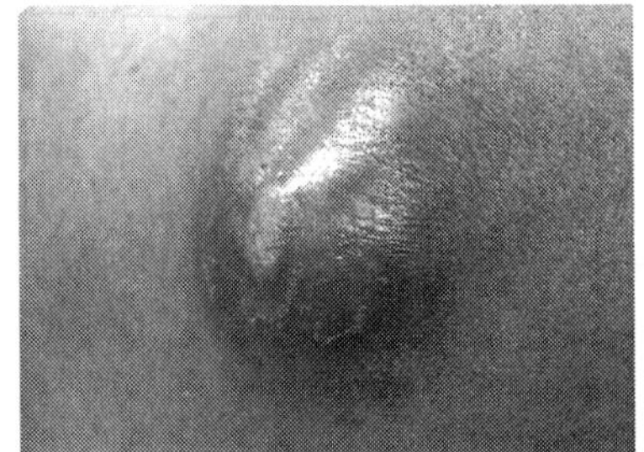

Abscess

If the abscess was not caused by an infected wound or diseased tooth, it is possible that it originated in a "**cyst**," which is a hollow structure filled with fluid. There are various types that can become infected and form abscesses:

- **Sebaceous Cysts**: skin glands often associated with hair follicles, they are concentrated on the face and trunk. These cysts produce oily material known as "sebum."
- **Inclusion Cysts**: These occur when skin lining is trapped in deeper layers as a result of trauma. During healing, they continue to produce skin cells and grow.
- **Pilonidal Cysts:** These cysts are located over the area of the tailbone, and are due to a malformation during fetal development. They easily become infected and require intervention.

With persistent abscesses, a route must be forged for the evacuation of pus. The easiest way to accomplish this is to place warm moist compresses over the area several times a day. This will help bring the infection to the surface of the skin, where it will form a "head" and perhaps drain spontaneously. This is called "ripening" the abscess. The abscess will go from firm to soft, and have a "whitehead" pimple at the likely point of exit.

Antibiotics like those mentioned for wound infection might help, but abscesses tend to be walled off by the immune system. These walls are difficult for medications like antibiotics to penetrate. If compresses and medications fail, you may have to intervene by performing a procedure called an "**incision and drainage**" ("I&D").

First, apply some ice or other anesthetic to the area to help numb the skin. Then, using the tip of a scalpel (a number 11 blade is best), pierce the skin over the abscess where it is closest to the surface. The pus should drain freely, and your patient will probably experience immediate relief from the release of pressure.

A gauze moistened with iodine tincture is then placed in the abscess cavity. Finally, apply some antibiotic ointment or raw unprocessed honey to the skin surrounding the incision and cover with a clean bandage. If the abscess returns, a more extensive surgical procedure may be necessary that removes the walls and some surrounding tissue.

Incision and drainage may be helpful for dental abscesses as well, but nearby teeth may still require extraction. A full discussion of dental disease and interventions is beyond the scope of this book, but can be found in The Survival Medicine Handbook: The Essential Guide for when Medical Help is Not on the Way.

Fungal Infections

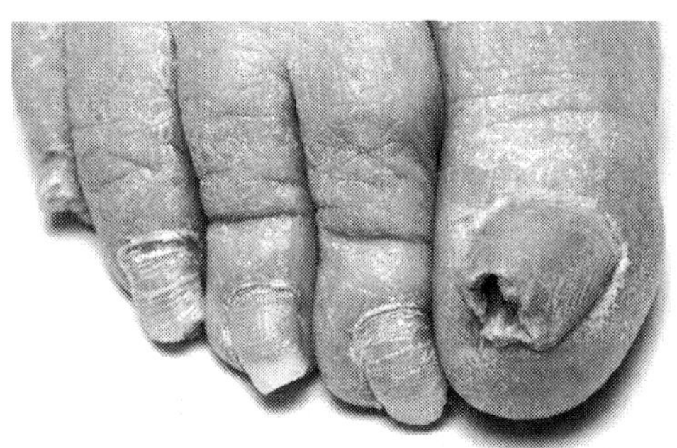

Severe fungal infection on toes

As the use of antibiotics to kill bacteria sometimes leads to secondary fungal infections, they should receive a mention here. Fungal infections are also known as "**mycoses**," and most often start in skin, lungs, oral cavity, or vagina. Skin infection with fungi was reported as the fourth most common disease in the world in 2010, affecting almost a billion people.

The areas of the skin most frequently affected include the feet, hands, nails, and scalp. These sites may exhibit fungal conditions like athlete's foot (also called "**tinea pedis**") and ringworm ("**tinea corporis**").

Fungal infections present as a reddish, sometimes raised, "flaky" rash with itching and burning. Toenails and fingernails may thicken and become yellow. More serious fungal infections in lungs and other internal organs are likely to be concentrated among the elderly and infirm.

Perhaps the most common vaginal infection is caused by the fungus Candida albicans. Although it is possible to transmit through intercourse, Candida is not considered to be a true sexually transmitted disease because it can occur in women who aren't sexually active. Overall, it is thought to affect 75% of all women at one point or another.

Symptoms include itching, burning, and a white or yellowish discharge with the consistency of "cottage cheese." Treatment involves the use of vaginal creams like miconazole or terconazole. Oral treatment with fluconazole is also acceptable and, indeed, preferred by many patients.

Examples of oral antifungal agents available in veterinary versions include the above-mentioned fluconazole as well as ketoconazole. A variety of topical creams and ointments are available for direct application to the skin such as clotrimazole. For the yeast infection called "**thrush**" that sometimes occurs in breastfeeding infants, an oral mouthwash called nystatin is effective.

TICK-BORNE DISEASES

Diseases transmitted by **vectors** like ticks, mosquitoes, and fleas have been taking their tolls on humans for thousands of years. Although mosquitoes transmit mostly viruses in the United States, ticks seem to transmit the most cases of bacterial disease. Due to encroaching civilization and other factors, many species have been extending their range throughout North America in recent years.

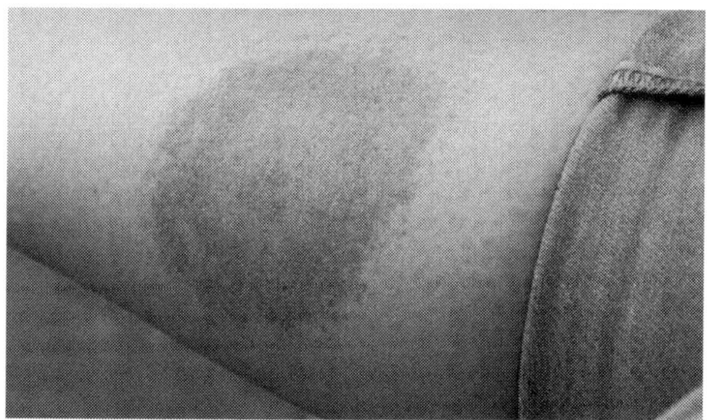

Erythema migrans rash in Lyme disease CROP

Lyme Disease

Lyme Disease, first identified in Old Lyme, Connecticut, is spread through the bite of ticks infected with the bacterium *Borrelia Burgdorferi*. Lyme disease infections occur on both U.S. coasts and follow the distribution of the deer tick, also called the blacklegged tick, and its western relatives. The distribution of this tick species (and others) has increased due to milder winters and larger deer populations.

Most humans are infected through the bites of juvenile ticks, called nymphs, so tiny that they're difficult to see. The adults can spread the disease but are more easily spotted and removed earlier. Lyme disease transmission usually doesn't occur until 24-48 hours after the bite; the faster you find the tick, the less likely you'll get the disease.

Lyme disease has a variety of signs and symptoms, some of which are seen in the first 2 or 3 weeks, and others that occur over months. The infection is diagnosed based on recognizing these symptoms, which is not always easy. Even trained medical professionals often miss the diagnosis.

Typical early symptoms include fever, headache, fatigue, and, often, a skin rash called **erythema migrans**. The rash looks remarkably like a bulls-eye that spreads out over time.

If left untreated, you can progress to chronic Lyme disease, where the infection can spread to joints, the heart, and the nervous system. You may see issues with swollen knees, loss of muscle tone, palpitations, irregular heartbeats, shortness of breath, nerve pain, numbness, and memory loss, every case seems to have its own subset of symptoms.

The antibiotics commonly used to treat Lyme disease include doxycycline and amoxicillin. Other antibiotic options include azithromycin and erythromycin. Early treatment is the key; later on, it becomes much more difficult to achieve a full recovery.

Rocky Mountain Spotted Fever

Rocky Mountain Spotted Fever is another tick-borne bacterial infection (there are at least 15 in the United States). The illness starts with a fever that occurs anywhere from 2-14 days after a tick bite. Several days later a rash appears which may be splotchy or pinpoint in appearance. Headache and other flu-like symptoms ensue.

Rocky Mountain Spotted Fever tends to damage blood vessels more than other tick-borne infections. Areas most affected are the extremities, especially fingers and toes. Damage may be so severe as to require amputation. Other long-term effects if untreated may include hearing loss, paralysis, or mental changes.

Unlike Lyme disease, the damage seems to done in the acute phase; no chronic stage has yet been reported. Early treatment with doxycycline or tetracycline is thought to be curative.

Other Tick-Borne Diseases

The Centers for Disease Control and Prevention reports more than 15 other diseases that are transmitted by tick bites in North America, including babesiosis, ehrlichiosis, anaplasmosis, Southern tick-associated rash illness, tick-borne relapsing fever, and tularemia. The pathogens are often bacteria, but parasites and viruses are also possibilities.

Although each illness has its own characteristics, symptoms you may see with the above diseases include:

- Body/muscle aches
- Fever
- Headaches
- Fatigue
- Joint pain
- Rash
- Stiff neck
- Facial paralysis

Although there is variation in treatment, clindamycin or doxycycline are often used, sometimes in conjunction with quinine, for babesiosis, ehrlichiosis, and others.

MENINGITIS

Meningitis is an inflammation of the protective membranes covering the brain and spinal cord, known as the "**meninges**." Meningitis can be caused by various pathogens, but most often viruses. Bacterial pathogens include *Neisseria meningitidis* (sometimes called "meningococcal meningitis"), *Streptococcus pneumoniae, Hemophilus influenzae* (type b), and others. The exact bacterial species seems to vary with the patient's age.

2-10 days after exposure, the patient with meningitis begins to experience a high fever, headache, and neck stiffness. As time progresses, symptoms like confusion, vomiting, and intolerance to light or sound manifest.

Very young children may appear irritable and lethargic without other specific symptoms. Infants 6 months or less with meningitis may be identified by the bulging of the soft spot (called the "**fontanelle**") on the top of the head.

Other signs of meningitis include the positive presence of **Kernig's sign** or **Brudzinski's sign**. Kernig's sign is assessed with the person lying supine, with the hip and knee flexed to 90 degrees. In a person with a positive Kernig's sign, pain limits passive extension of the knee. A positive Brudzinski's sign occurs when flexion of the neck causes involuntary flexion of the knee and hip.

Meningitis due to *Neisseria meningitidis* ("meningococcal meningitis") can be differentiated from other types by a rash consisting of small, irregular purple or red spots called "**petechiae**." These spots, which don't blanch when pressure is applied, can be found on the trunk, lower extremities, conjunctiva, and mucous membranes.

Failure to treat meningitis is likely fatal due to increased pressure in the brain, seizures, sepsis, and spontaneous bleeding due to depletion of clotting factors.

Intravenous therapy with benzylpenicillin, vancomycin, or ceftriaxone is considered reasonable empirical therapy; oral antibiotics like ciprofloxacin may have a role in preventing spread to family members. Survivors of meningitis infections often have long-term ill effects, such as hearing loss or mental deficits.

DENTAL INFECTIONS

In any austere setting (at least where there is a source of sugar), dental infections are likely to run rampant in the community. As the healthcare provider, you will certainly be asked to evaluate and treat issues relating to teeth. Many of these will relate to infection.

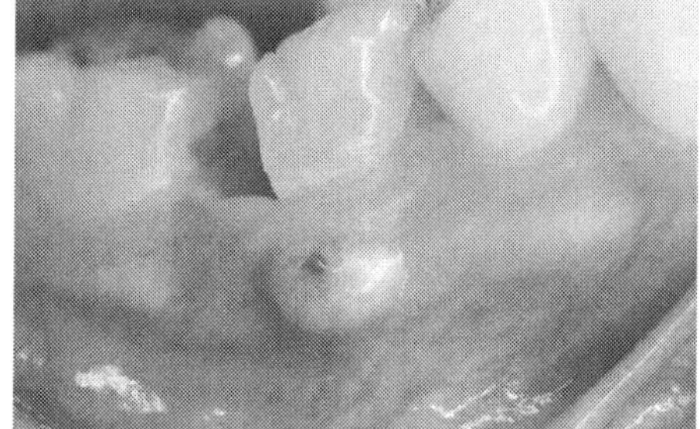

Dental abscess

There are several dental infections that can cause significant pain and tooth loss. Every aspect of tooth anatomy, from the hard, shiny enamel to the deep pulp tissue, can be damaged by bacteria. For example, streptococcal infection may cause tooth decay that invades all the way down to the root of the tooth. Strep and Staph infections may affect the soft tissue around the tooth, forming a collection of pus called an **abscess**. Bacteria like *Porphyromonas gingivalis* may infect the gums, causing a condition called "**gingivitis**."

Possible symptoms of tooth infections include:

- Toothache
- Sensitivity to hot and/or cold
- Pain when chewing
- Foul taste

- Fever
- Bad breath
- Red, swollen gums
- Open sores
- Swollen lymph nodes under the jaw and in the neck

Antibiotics in the penicillin and cephalosporin families are favored by dentists to treat many dental infections. If allergic to penicillin, metronidazole may be used.

Tooth abscesses must also often be surgically drained. Although the goal of modern dentistry is to salvage every tooth, extraction may be the treatment of choice off the grid for any infection that fails to respond to antibiotic therapy. Description of various dental procedures, including extraction, can be found in either "The Survival Medicine Handbook: The Essential Guide for When Medical Help is Not on the Way" or the venerable "Where There is No Dentist."

BACTERIAL INFECTIONS THAT WILL BECOME COMMON

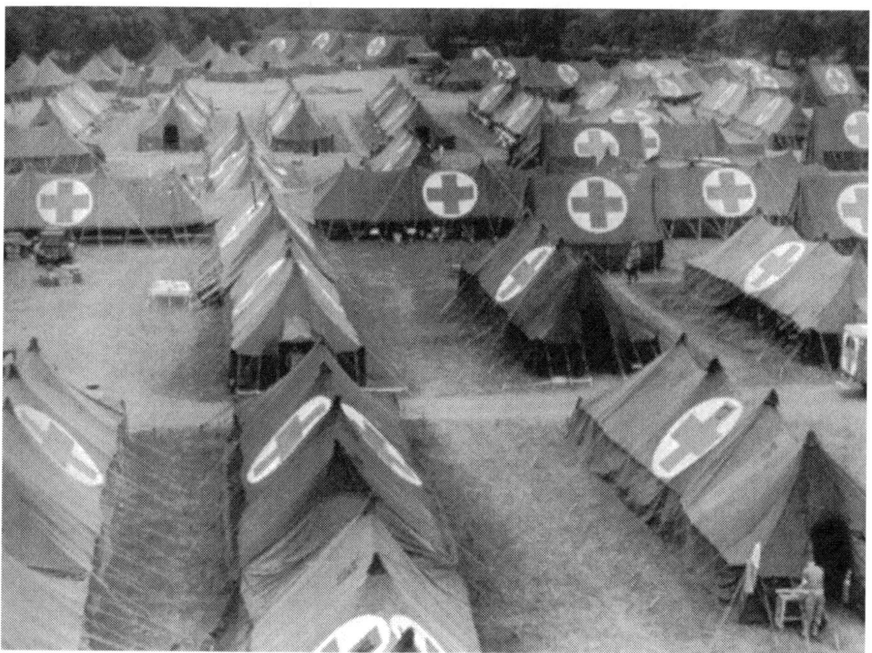

The infectious diseases below sometimes came in waves of epidemics in years past, but are rare in developed countries today. In the United States, improved sanitation and modern medical facilities have gone a long way towards eliminating illnesses like cholera and malaria.

It's important to understand, however, that many of the bacterial and parasitic diseases below are quite common in austere locations where modern medicine and antibiotics are scarce commodities. A major event that takes away access to high technology will give an opportunity for many of these infections to take root even in the most advanced society.

Cholera

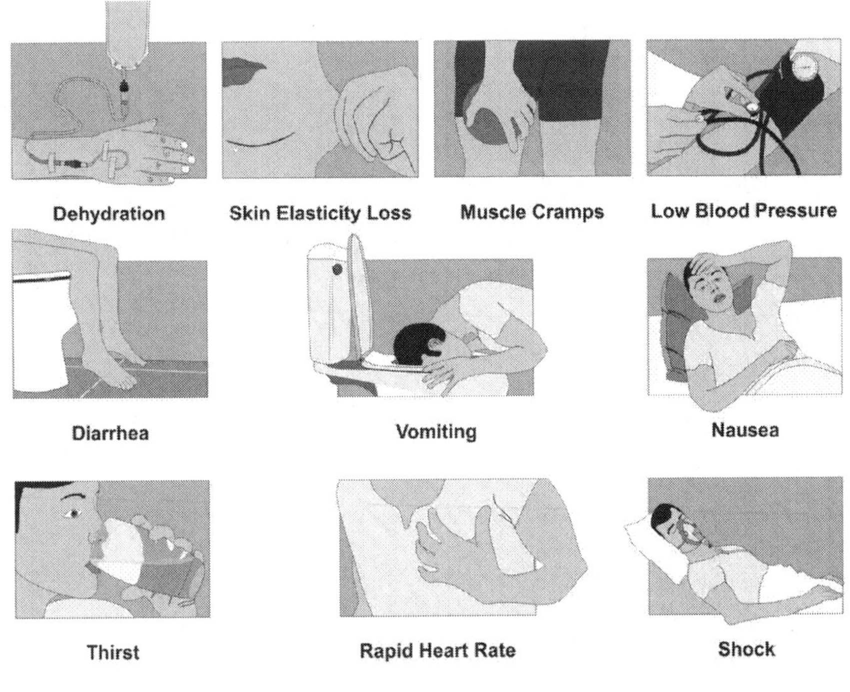

Cholera symptoms

Caused by the marine and freshwater bacterium *Vibrio cholerae*, cholera has been reported as a pandemic outbreak seven times since the 1800s. Even in modern times, millions of cases have been reported worldwide, including in the aftermath of the 2011 earthquake in Haiti. Indeed, a cholera epidemic is raging in Zimbabwe as this book was being written.

Cholera toxins produce a rapid onset of diarrhea, vomiting, and leg cramps within a few hours to 2 days of infection. The water loss with untreated cholera is so rapid and severe that sixty per cent of victims perish. Bowel movements look very much like the water left in a pot after boiling rice, giving them the name "rice-water stools."

Aggressive efforts to rehydrate the patient, especially intravenously, helps counteract the severe water loss experienced and drops the death rate to one per cent. A recipe for homemade oral rehydration solution is described later in this book. Antibiotic therapy with doxycycline or tetracycline seems to shorten the duration of illness.

Typhus

A complex of diseases caused by bacteria in the *Rickettsia* family, typhus can be transmitted by body lice, fleas, or ticks to humans. Each type varies somewhat with the insect that carries it. In general, typhus poses a risk in any situation where there are issues with hygiene and sanitation.

In the past, typhus was a common source of epidemics in the wake of wars and famines. Typhus was first noted at the Spanish siege of Granada in 1482-1492, where 3,000 Spaniards died in combat but 17,000 succumbed to the disease. It is thought that more of Napoleon's soldiers died of typhus in their 1812 retreat from Moscow than were killed by Russians. More recently, many in German concentration camps died of the infection, including the 15-year-old Anne Frank. Conversely, large numbers of German prisoners of war in WWII Russian prison camps were victims of the disease.

Although it rarely causes severe diarrhea, Typhus can cause dehydration due to high fevers and other flu-like symptoms which start one to two weeks after exposure. Five to nine days later, a rash begins on the torso and spreads to the back and extremities. Upon examination, you will find that the rash spares the face, palm, and soles. If untreated, sores can form that become **necrotic** and death rates approach 20 percent. Doxycycline is the drug of choice for this disease. Treated, the death rate drops to less than one percent.

Typhoid Fever

Salmonella typhi is a bacterium found in contaminated and undercooked food and water. The illness it causes is called "Typh-oid fever" because it is often confused with Typhus. Food poisoning with Salmonella occurs more often than with any other bacteria in the United States. The CDC reports that there are 22 million cases reported worldwide every year.

In Typhoid fever, there is an incubation period averaging 8-14 days. After a gradual onset of high fevers over several days, abdominal pain, intestinal hemorrhage, weakness, headaches, constipation, and bloody diarrhea may occur. A number of people develop a spotty, rose-colored rash.

Typhoid fever seems to appear in four week-long stages:

Stage 1: The patient develops a high fever peaking in the afternoon, along with cough and headache. Some experience bleeding from the nose. A drop in the heart rate (**bradycardia**) is noted, which is an unusual finding in someone with fever. Normally, a patient with a fever has a high heart rate (**tachycardia**).

Stage 2: Fever remains elevated, and, if untreated, the patient becomes delirious. Rose-colored spots appear on the lower chest and abdomen in around a third of patients. Foul-smelling green diarrhea that is reminiscent of pea soup is often seen in this stage. Weight loss occurs as the abdomen becomes distended due to an enlarged liver and spleen.

Stage 3: Damage to the intestines leads to bleeding or perforation of the wall. An infection of blood called "**septicemia**" occurs and the lining of the abdomen becomes inflamed ("**peritonitis**"). Blood clotting factors become depleted which may lead to more bleeding. The patient's mental status worsens. 12-30 percent of untreated sufferers don't survive beyond this point.

Stage 4: Fever slowly reduces in those that survive to the fourth week, but intestinal and mental effects may persist for months. The victim looks emaciated and may still harbor the organism as a "**carrier**."

Ciprofloxacin is the antibiotic of choice; Azithromycin is another alternative. Survival rate is greater than 99 percent in treated populations.

Dysentery

Dysentery is an intestinal inflammation in the large intestine that presents with fever, abdominal pain, and severe bloody or watery mucus diarrhea. Symptoms usually begin one to three days after exposure. A major cause of death among Civil War soldiers, dysentery is a classic example of a disease that can be prevented with strict hand hygiene after bowel movements.

The most common form of dysentery in North America and Europe is caused by the bacteria *Shigella*. It is more commonly called "bacillary dysentery." Both are spread through contaminated food and water in crowded, unsanitary conditions. Ciprofloxacin and Sulfa drugs, in conjunction with oral rehydration, are effective therapies.

Entamoeba histolytica, an organism sometimes classified as a protozoan, is another possible cause of dysentery. Also known as "amebiasis" or "amoebic dysentery," it appears 2-4 weeks after exposure and appears much like bacillary dysentery. Failure to treat early with antibiotics like Metronidazole or Tinidazole may cause long-term organ damage.

Tetanus

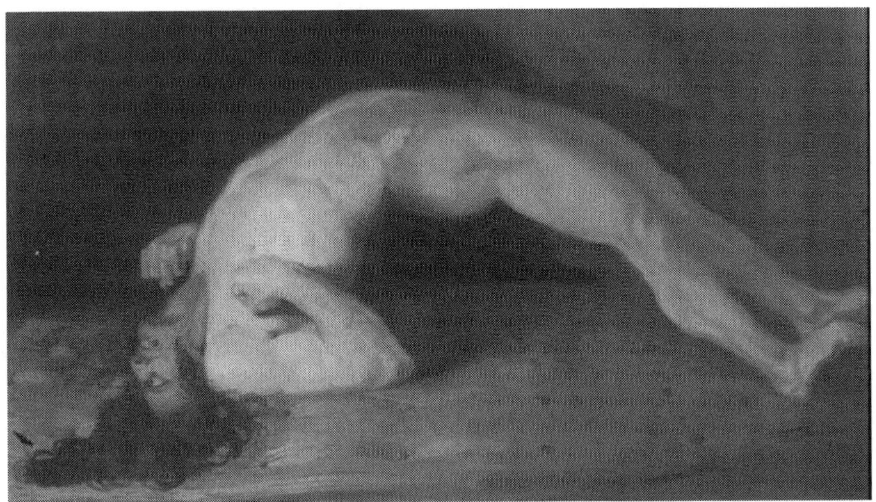

Muscle spasms seen in full-blown tetanus infection

Tetanus (from the Greek word *tetanos*, meaning tight) is an infection caused by the bacterium *Clostridium tetani*. The bacteria produce **spores** that primarily live in the soil or the feces of animals. These spores are capable of laying dormant for years and are resistant to extremes in temperature.

Most tetanus infections occur when a person has experienced a break in the skin. The skin is the body's armor; any defect in it leaves a person open to infection. The most common cause is some type of puncture wound, such as an insect or animal bite, a splinter, or even a rusty nail (or, for that matter, a non-rusty nail).

Puncture wounds are more likely to harbor tetanus because the bacterium is **anaerobic**. That means that it doesn't like oxygen; deep, narrow wounds like punctures give less access to it. Any injury that compromises the skin, however, is eligible.

When a wound becomes contaminated with Tetanus spores, the spore becomes activated as a full-fledged bacterium and reproduces rapidly. Damage to the victim comes as a result of a strong toxin excreted by the organism known as Tetanospasmin. This toxin specifically targets nerves that serve muscle tissue, causing "misfires" that lead to involuntary contractions. These symptoms are often combined with fever, elevated blood pressure, and difficulty swallowing.

Effects can be localized or affect the entire body. After an incubation period of 1-2 weeks, you would possibly see the classical symptom of "**Lockjaw**," where the jaw muscle becomes taut. A spasmodic arching of the back may be seen in other cases. Any muscle group exposed to the toxin is susceptible, including those used in breathing.

Early treatment is vital and may consist of Metronidazole or Doxycycline.

Malaria

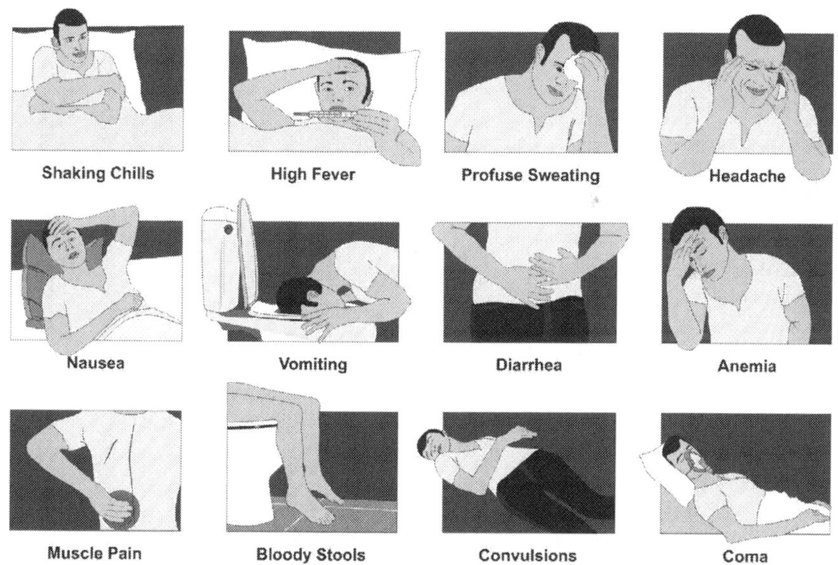

Symptoms of malaria

Malaria, a protozoan disease transmitted by mosquitoes, is the cause of many deaths in the underdeveloped world, and was an issue in the United States until the introduction of the pesticide DDT. Even today, The World Health Organization reports 300-500 million cases every year.

Malaria is caused by one of four species of microbe called "plasmodium," of which *Plasmodium falciparum* seems to be the worst. Plasmodium lives in the gut of mosquitoes. When an anopheles species mosquito injects plasmodium into a human body, it colonizes organs such as the liver. Once there, the parasite travels through your circulation to damage blood cells and other organs.

Symptoms of Malaria appear 10-28 days after exposure and seem flu-like in nature. The victim may present with periodic chills, fever, and sweats. The classic appearance includes:

- High fever (often reaching 104 degrees Fahrenheit or more)
- Shaking chills
- Extreme sweating
- Fatigue
- Joint and body aches
- Headache
- Nausea and vomiting
- Diarrhea

Some of the worst cases develop jaundice, a yellowing of the skin and eyes due to liver damage. Untreated malaria is often episodic, with relapses that come closer and closer together as time progresses.

The medications used for Malaria include Chloroquine, Quinine, and Quinidine; other, later-generation drugs, are also available. Sometimes, an antibiotic such as Doxycycline or Clindamycin is used in combination with the above. A study at malariajournal.biomedcentral.com suggests that the sulfa drug combo Sulfamethoxazole/Trimethoprim may have potential in malaria treatment and others (mentioned later) may be useful in prevention.

Tuberculosis

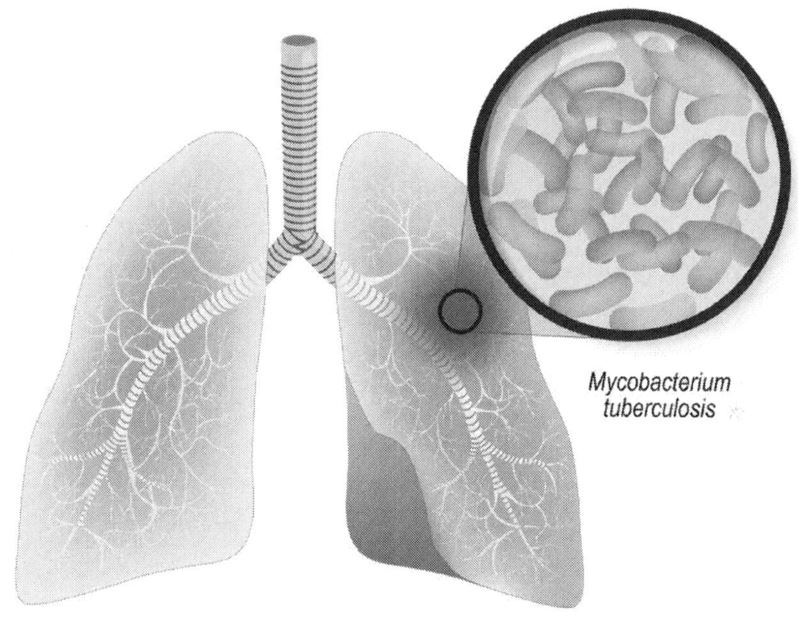

Tuberculosis

Tuberculosis is a contagious disease caused by the bacterium called *Mycobacterium tuberculosis*. Spread by air droplets, it is most commonly associated with the lungs but can affect various organs. The disease is so prevalent in underdeveloped countries that it is thought that total cases number over one billion. In 2010, 1.5 million deaths were associated with the infection.

Primary tuberculosis (known as "**latent**" TB) does not cause symptoms, so it is often missed by medical professionals in its early stages. When symptoms become apparent (sometimes years later), TB is said to have become "active."

Symptoms of active tuberculosis in the lungs include:

- Cough, sometimes painful, that lasts for more than three weeks
- Blood in the sputum
- Chest pain, especially with breathing

- Weight loss
- Fever and chills
- Night sweats
- Loss of appetite

Over time, the victim loses so much weight that the disease appears to be consuming them. As such, tuberculosis was known as "**consumption**." Progression of the disease leads to severe damage of the organs affected.

Although tuberculosis is contagious through air droplets from coughs and sneezes, it is most likely to be caught from someone with whom you are in close contact. Treatment consists of several antibiotics in combination which must be taken for months. Once treated for two weeks or more, however, the patient is usually no longer contagious.

There are strains of TB reported to show significant resistance to the usual combination of drugs. These are called "multiple drug-resistant" or MDR Tuberculosis. Treating these cases is a major challenge even in the age of modern medicine.

Anthrax

Anthrax is a disease caused by *Bacillus anthracis* that can take several forms. It may affect the lungs, intestines, or skin; each variation has its own set of symptoms. Anthrax has become a major concern for its potential use as a bioterror agent. Anthrax has incredible longevity in adverse conditions: Its inactive form (called a "**spore**") is extremely hardy and may survive for several decades in the soil.

Cutaneous anthrax: 95% of anthrax infections are "**cutaneous**"; that is, they affect the skin. Contact with infected soil or livestock may cause the infection. With cutaneous anthrax, you may see a raised itchy bump or blister at first. This progresses to a painless skin ulcer with a center area of black, **necrotic** tissue. This usually occurs anywhere from 1 to 7 days after exposure to the organism. Untreated, cutaneous anthrax has a 20% death rate.

Gastrointestinal anthrax: Intestinal anthrax may affect the GI tract if the victim consumes contaminated meat. Symptoms include loss of appetite, fever, nausea, vomiting of blood, and bloody diarrhea. Expect a death rate of 25-60 per cent.

Respiratory anthrax: Also called "inhalational anthrax," this version is usually brought on by breathing in spores from infected animal products (or bioterror gases). Symptoms begin 1-7 days after exposure but may start later.

At first, inhalational anthrax resembles a simple cold, but after several days, the patient begins to experience fever, chest pain, and breathing difficulty due to fluid accumulation in the lungs. This leads to respiratory failure and shock. Respiratory anthrax is commonly fatal.

Fortunately, anthrax is not generally contagious from human to human. Antibiotics that are effective if used early in the disease include ciprofloxacin, doxycycline, and penicillin.

Plague

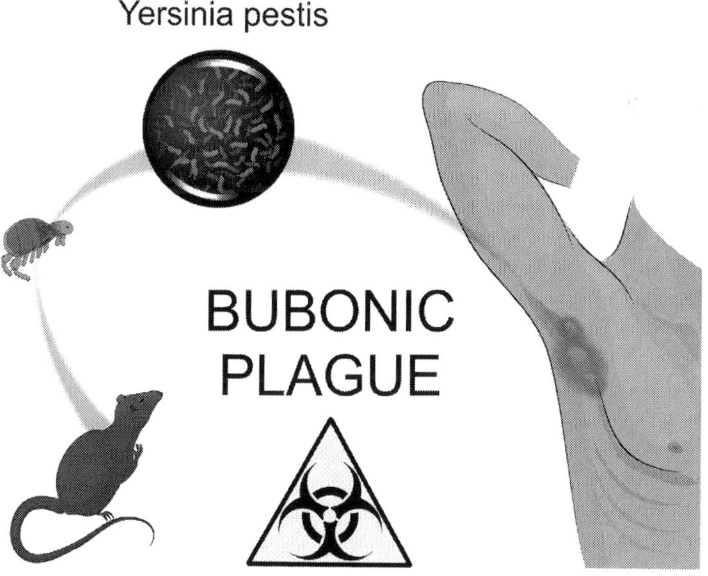

Plague, once called "The Black Death," is caused by the bacteria *Yersinia pestis*, a bacterium found in fleas that infest rats and other rodents. The infection is transmitted from animal to animal (or human) when infected fleas latch onto and bite a new host.

Like anthrax, there are several types of Plague. Once established, different forms of plague can be spread by air droplets from coughs, in the blood, or even by contaminated water or food. They are:

Bubonic plague: The most common type, bubonic plague has an incubation period of 2-6 days before it causes fever, chills, and other flu-like symptoms. Later, it causes an accumulation of bacteria, blood, and pus in lymph nodes. These become painful, swollen lumps called "**buboes**." Buboes turn black in color and may be seen in the armpits, groin, and neck.

Other symptoms include vomiting of blood, gastrointestinal issues, breathing difficulty, seizures, and **gangrene** (loss of circulation) to the extremities such as toes, fingers, nose, and lips. Untreated, death occurs in a week to ten days.

Pneumonic plague: Pneumonic plague infects the lungs and can develop in those with bubonic plague or who breathe in infected air droplets. Within one to three days after exposure, the victim begins to cough up blood (also known as "**hemoptysis**") and develops chest pain and shortness of breath. If untreated, death occurs in less than 48 hours.

Septicemic plague: Bacteria may pass from buboes to poison the bloodstream, or may directly enter the body through an open wound. Besides fever and other general symptoms, a depletion in blood clotting factors may cause spontaneous and unstoppable bleeding into the skin, lungs, kidneys, and other organs.

Antibiotics combined with supportive therapy like hydration are effective against plague *if* patients are diagnosed in time. Doxycycline, Tetracycline, or Ciprofloxacin may be good choices for therapy.

Diphtheria

Diphtheria is a highly contagious inflammation of the mucous membranes caused by a toxin produced by the Gram-positive bacteria *Corynebacterium diphtheriae.*

Classically, Diphtheria forms a grey or white patch in the throat about 2-5 days after exposure that is accompanied by sore throat, fever, and cough. Sometimes, swelling in the neck occurs due to swollen glands that causes difficulty breathing. Other features include a skin rash that resembles impetigo and signs of nerve and heart damage.

Diphtheria treatment involves the use of an antitoxin and antibiotics. The Centers for Disease Control and Prevention recommends metronidazole, erythromycin, or clindamycin. Due to vaccination programs, diphtheria is rare outside of underdeveloped countries.

Necrotizing Fasciitis

Mentioned briefly above, necrotizing fasciitis is a soft-tissue infection that rapidly spreads and can be extremely dangerous. It can be caused by various bacterial species including strep, staph/MRSA, and enterococci species, but also in infections with bacteria like *Clostridia* or *Vibrio vulnificus*. Whatever the causative agent, you will see it reported as "flesh-eating bacteria."

Necrotizing infections can occur when bacteria enter wounds. Fisherman may get Vibrio vulnificus, for example, as a result of puncture wounds from fish spines or hooks. It often appears within a day as a blistering skin infection. As time goes on, fever develops as the infection spreads.

Early symptoms appear like the flu. The course of the disease is so rapid that the victim is severely ill by the time they are first seen by medical personnel. These patients have significant fever, diarrhea, swelling, and bloody blisters called "**bullae**."

Tissue death occurs in various locations which requires the cutting away of affected tissue through a process called "**debridement**." The death rate depends on the speed of correct diagnosis and aggressiveness of management, but ranges from 33-75% once the infection spreads to the blood.

Antibiotics like clindamycin may be effective, dependent on the extent of the infection. Older or **immune-compromised** individuals are most severely affected and have the worst **prognosis**.

Botulism

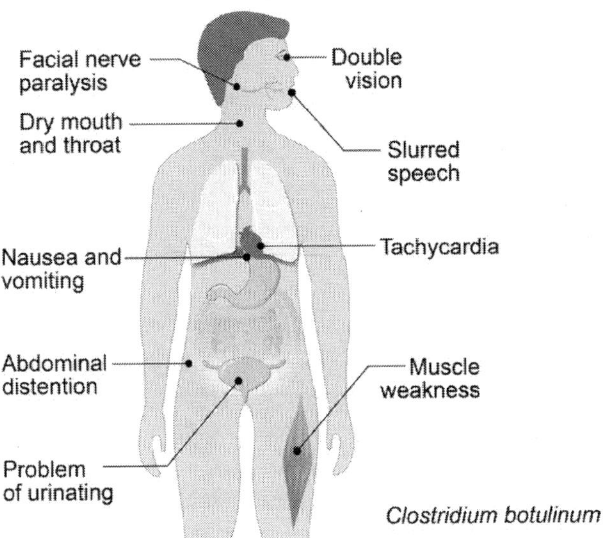

Symptoms of botulism

Botulism is caused by toxins produced by the anaerobic bacterium *Clostridium botulinum*. Infection occurs as a result of eating contaminated food or from a deep puncture wound. Botulism is also sometimes present in honey, a good reason why it is forbidden to feed infants under 12 months.

Beginning 12-72 hours after exposure, symptoms begin which involve nerves, starting with the face. The victim experiences difficulty with facial muscles, eye movements, chewing, swallowing. The patient may exhibit drooping eyelids and complain of double vision.

As the disease progresses, the patient loses strength in muscles of the torso and extremities. Intestinal symptoms may also occur, such as diarrhea, nausea and vomiting, and abdominal swelling. As nerve damage progresses, constipation occurs as the intestines shut down. Interestingly, fever is rarely present.

Antibiotics (Penicillin G or metronidazole) may be effective in botulism due to wound contamination, but an **antitoxin** is given in most instances. It is preferred because killing the bacteria with antibiotics releases more toxins as they die. A 5-10% **mortality rate** is expected.

Leprosy (Hansen's Disease)

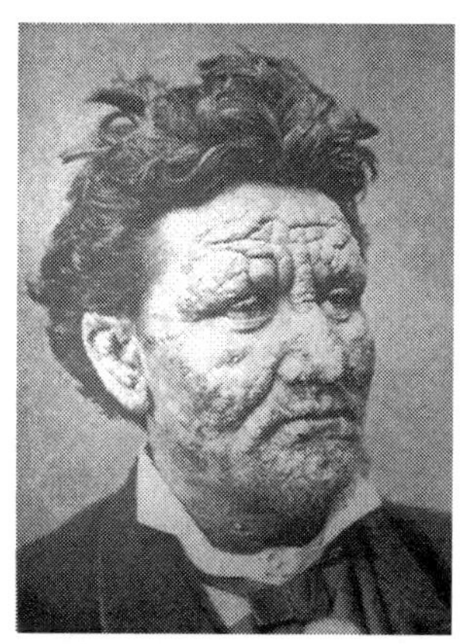

Leprosy (now called "Hansen's Disease") is considered a disease of the past, but the bacterial infection continues to be reported today in the Southern United States. Experts suggest that the armadillo may be a vector; they are a "**reservoir**" for the bacteria *Mycobacterium leprae* that causes the disease. Hansen's Disease is the second most common disease caused by mycobacteria after tuberculosis.

The **incubation period** for Hansen's disease can be up to 10 years (average 2-3 years), making it very difficult to identify the original source of exposure.

Despite victims being cast out from society in the past, leprosy is actually not that contagious. You can catch it only if you come into frequent contact with droplets from coughs and sneezes from someone who has it. In addition, a percentage of the population seems, for unknown reasons, to be immune.

Leprosy primarily affects the skin, where the first signs usually occur. It also affects the nerves outside the brain and spinal cord, called the "peripheral" nerves. It may also involve the eyes, the lining of the nose, the kidneys, and even male sexual organs.

Over time, nerve damage causes sufferers to experience loss of sensation to these areas. People with advanced disease may lose their fingers, toes, and nose. Muscle weakness and paralysis can also occur, leading to claw-like deformities of the hands and difficulty walking.

People can also get Hansen's disease through their circulatory system. When that happens, the bacterium slowly infiltrates the tissues under the skin, and causes sores, pale bumps and skin protuberances on the face. This can lead to unusual features, in which the infected develop an enlarged brow and cheekbone features.

Today, Hansen's disease is treatable with 6 months to 2 years of multiple antibiotic therapies. Despite this, an estimated 2 million people are thought to suffer from the infection in underdeveloped countries. From a practical standpoint, the supplies of antibiotics available would be insufficient to help victims of this illness in a long-term disaster.

HOW TO TELL BACTERIAL VS. VIRAL DISEASE

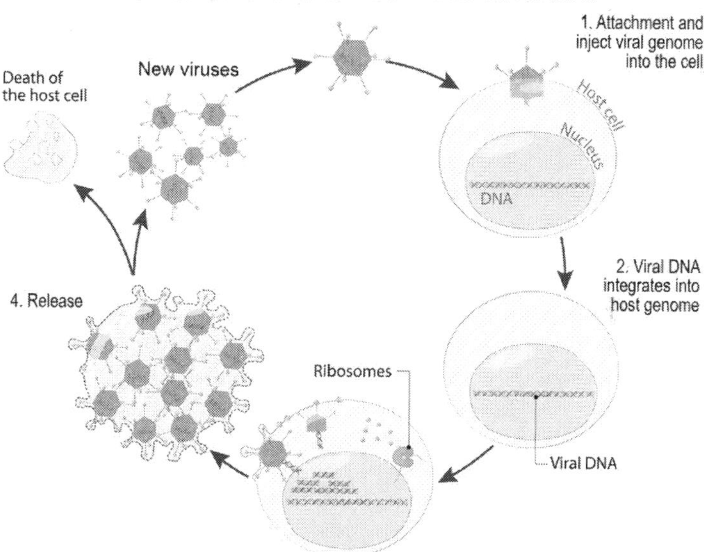

Today, we have advanced laboratory studies that allow identification of many pathogens. Despite this, it can be a challenge for healthcare providers to tell a bacterial disease from a viral one. Bacteria and virus can attack the same organ systems.

For example, **pneumonia** can be bacterial or viral. Both produce similar symptoms like cough and fever. From a diagnosis standpoint, it can be difficult to tell the difference even in normal times.

In disaster settings, it's worse; there's a limited supply of medicines that can't be replaced. An antibiotic would have no effect on a viral infection. To waste precious antibiotics on a virus may be catastrophic for the next person with a legitimate bacterial infection.

What can a caregiver without access to modern facilities do to distinguish between a bacterial and a viral infection?

Although bacteria and viruses are both microscopic organisms that can cause disease, they are as alike as a bullfrog and a blue whale. There are major differences in structure and, although subtler, in their symptoms.

Bacteria are single-celled creatures with a rigid wall and a membrane surrounding the cell. Viruses aren't even a cell; they consist only of some genetic material held together by a coat of protein. Viruses are much smaller than bacteria but outnumber them ten to one.

Bacteria can reproduce on their own without the aid of a host. Viruses must enter a host cell and use it as a factory to manufacture new viruses. They accomplish this by changing the host's genetic material from normal functions to multiplying the virus.

Most bacteria are harmless; less than one percent are pathogenic. Viruses, on the other hand, often cause disease. They can even target bacteria as a host. Viruses do this so often that an article in Nature magazine claims they kill half of the world's bacteria every two days.

What can a caregiver without access to modern facilities do to tell the difference between a bacterial and a viral infection? Some subtle differences might point you in the right direction:

- The length of the illness. Many viral infections are self-limited; they improve on their own (if they don't kill the host, that is). Most show significant improvement by 10 days or so. Bacterial infections, if untreated, may last much longer.
- The severity of fevers. Bacterial infections tend to be associated with impressive temperature spikes. Viral infections may or may not show a tendency to cause fever. What is considered a fever? Standard medical wisdom considers a fever to be 38 degrees Centigrade (100.4 degrees Fahrenheit), but patients usually feel sick above 37 degrees Centigrade (more than 99 degrees Fahrenheit)

- The color of the mucus. In viral respiratory infections, the phlegm is usually whitish or clear. Mucus may be yellow or green in bacterial infections.
- **Localized** or **systemic**? Viral have more tendency to cause widespread symptoms, while bacterial infections may be local in nature.
- Pimples and white spots: Pimples on the skin or white spots on the back of the throat or tonsils are generally caused by bacteria.
- Are there any other symptoms? A sore throat without a runny nose or sneezing may be a bacterial infection such as strep throat.

It should be noted that there are many exceptions to the above.

Sometimes, bacteria might invade a patient weakened by a viral illness. This is called a "secondary infection" and makes its presence known by a sudden "turn for the worse" after a period of apparent improvement. Making a definitive diagnosis is often a challenge.

Infections in certain parts of the body may be more likely to be bacterial:

- Urinary Tract Infections
- Wound Infections
- Skin infections (may also be fungal)
- Soft tissue infections
- Abscesses

Respiratory infections may be caused by bacteria or viruses, but once in the lung itself, the percentage chance it is bacterial increases.

SECTION 3

+++

BASICS OF ANTIBIOTICS

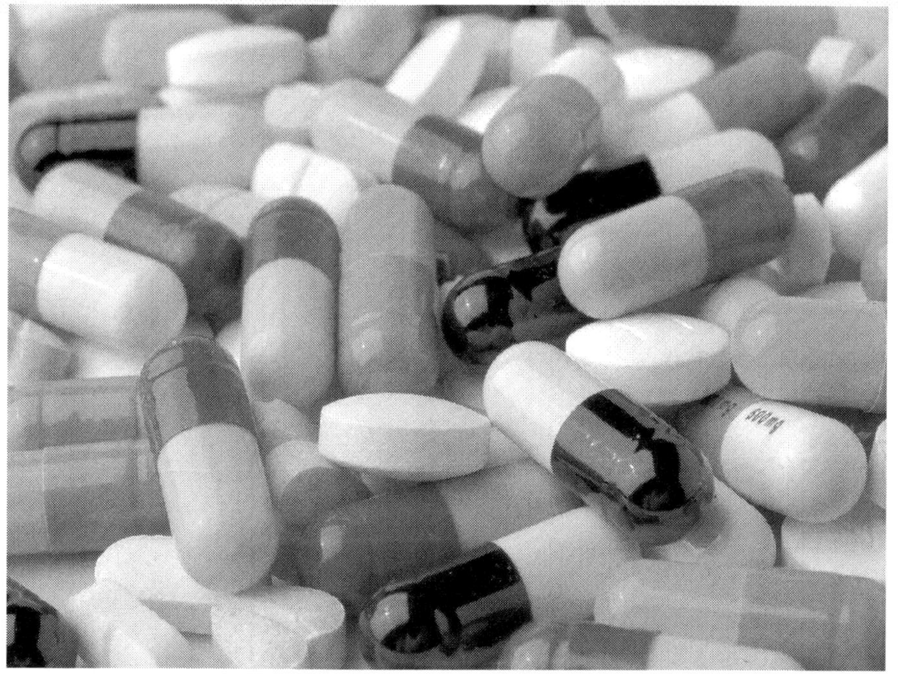

WHAT ARE ANTIBIOTICS?

What are antibiotics and why do we benefit from their existence?

The human body is a marvel of biologic engineering on many levels. Our immune system kills harmful germs before they can multiply and cause symptoms. Our blood contains white cells, also known as "**leukocytes**," that attack pathogens.

Even if we do experience symptoms, our bodies usually cope and fight off the infection. Although we don't realize it's happening, this process of exposure to infection and its elimination by normal immune response is a daily occurrence.

There are occasions, however, when the body's defenses are overwhelmed. In these cases, intervention is required. It comes in the form of **antibiotics**. Antibiotics are medicines that kill bacterial and, sometimes, other infections. The word "antibiotics" is derived from the Greek "anti" ("against") and "bios" ("life"). While this seems a strange origin for a medicine that saves lives, the meaning is simply that the drug is "against" the life of the disease-causing organism.

There are a number of terms for substances that cure infections. Antimicrobials is a general term for anything that kills microbes. The common use of the term antibiotic implies action against bacteria but may include certain protozoa or fungi. Perhaps more specific terms would be antibacterial, antifungal, or anti-protozoal drugs. We'll use the common usage of the term antibiotic, however, in this book.

Note that we didn't include "anti-viral drugs" in the above paragraph. Antibiotics work to inhibit protein synthesis or reproduction of bacteria, but the anatomy of viruses is very different. To think antibiotics would work against viruses is like expecting diesel gasoline to power a starship.

That said, antibiotics are powerful medicines that fight certain infections and can even stop epidemics when used properly. Each medication eliminates bacterial populations in various ways, ranging from outright destruction to the inhibition of the germ's ability to repair itself or reproduce.

A SHORT HISTORY OF ANTIBIOTICS

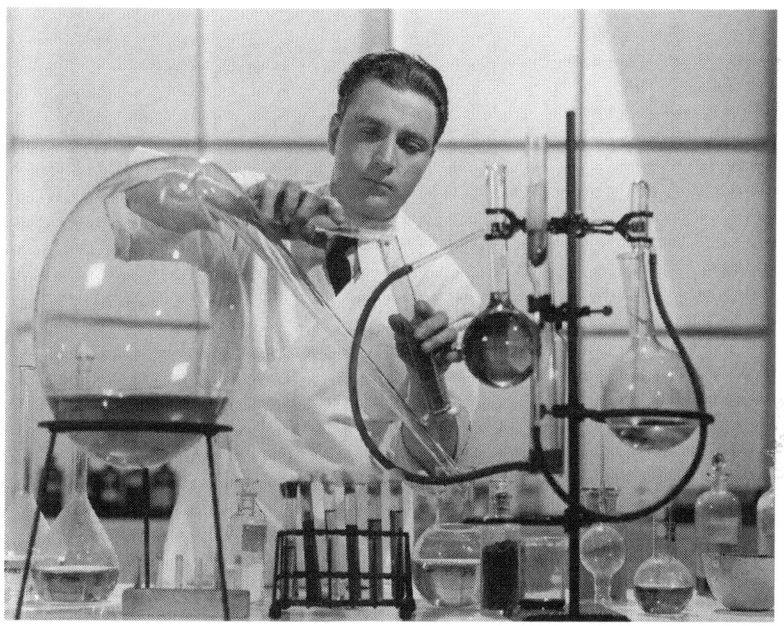

Discovery of certain antibiotics were surprises.

Although ancient cultures were unaware of the microscopic germs that cause infections, many developed and used treatments to deal with the sicknesses caused by them. In some instances, they utilized the very raw materials that became the basis for modern antibiotics like penicillin.

The earliest known evidence of antibiotics has been found in chemical analyses of the bones of ancient Nubians, a civilization that lived in what is now Sudan (South of Egypt) two thousand years ago. Studies on the remains of these people suggested the ingestion of the antibiotic tetracycline on a regular basis. How was this possible? Finding tetracycline, a drug first introduced in modern times after World War II, in relics that old is tantamount to finding a Neanderthal skeleton holding a cell phone!

After some understandable skepticism on the part of the scientific community, it was proposed that the Nubians accidentally produced the tetracycline when they made beer. The antibiotic is produced by a bacterium in the soil that grows well in hot, dry areas such as Egypt and Sudan. Likely, it contaminated the beer during the fermentation process.

To test this theory, graduate students experimented with making the beer and, sure enough, it had tetracycline in it (although it didn't look much like beer, honestly).

The result of the accidental intake of the antibiotics was that the remains of the ancient Nubians didn't seem to show much evidence of infection. Reports of Egyptian skeletons from the same era or earlier also seemed to contained evidence of tetracycline in their bones and were relatively free of disease.

Fast forward to modern times: The first officially-recognized antibiotic that was discovered for the cure of infection may actually be a matter for discussion. The answer may lie in, of all things, blue cheese. The Chinese and Indian cultures used molds in the cure of disease, but with little idea how they worked. In 1874, a physician named William Roberts noted that a mold called Penicillium glaucum, utilized in the making of blue cheese, seemed to prevent the growth of bacteria in lab dishes. Sometime later, the noted scientist Louis Pasteur showed similar results with anthrax bacteria by using a related Penicillium mold.

While the discovery of the connection between molds and bacterial inhibition was important, it didn't result, at the time, in a product that could be released to the general public.

Meanwhile, German scientist Paul Ehrlich was experimenting with dyes in the 1880s. He proposed that it was possible to make chemicals from the dyes that would kill bacteria without harming the human body. On his 606th attempt in 1907, he discovered the first synthetic antibacterial agent, an arsenic compound now called arsphenamine. It was used as early as 1910 to treat the sexually transmitted disease known as syphilis.

It wasn't until 1927, however, that Scottish physician and microbiologist Alexander Fleming discovered a usable antibiotic from molds. Amazingly, it was by accident.

It seems that Dr. Fleming's laboratory was somewhat untidy. In August of 1927, Fleming left a number of bacterial specimens out when he took a family vacation. Returning the next month, he noticed that one of them had developed a fungus. Strangely, the bacterial colonies surrounding the fungus were gone.

Fleming identified the fungus as being from the Penicillium family, as had been previously discovered by Roberts and Pasteur. He called his discovery "mold juice" until it was officially named penicillin in 1929. Further investigation on penicillin's effect on bacteria revealed that it inhibited various types, including the germs that caused scarlet fever, diphtheria, meningitis, and certain pneumonias.

Despite this, Fleming couldn't find a way to mass produce his new discovery; that was left to Drs. Howard Florey and Ernst Boris Chain in Oxford, England. They took up further research with financial aid from the United States and Great Britain. When another researcher, Dr. Howard Heatley, made a breakthrough in purifying the final product, they started mass production.

This was fortunate timing, as penicillin became available to the public just after the bombing of Pearl Harbor. Half of the total supply was used on the first patient in early 1942. The antibiotic was considered so useful, however, that by 1945, 646 billion doses were manufactured annually.

From these crude beginnings, many penicillin-related antibiotics were developed and are widely used today to treat a variety of infections.

You might think that Penicillin was the first drug to achieve wide market appeal, but it was preceded by another popular family of antibiotics called sulfonamides. These became widely-available in the 1930s.

Indeed, Sulfa drugs have been called "the first miracle drug." They deserve credit for saving tens of thousands of lives during World War Two, including those of Winston Churchill and the son of Franklin Delano Roosevelt. It was so widely used early in the war that many soldiers' first aid kits often came with the drug in pill or powder form. Medics were instructed to pour it into any open wound.

THE PERFECT ANTIBIOTIC

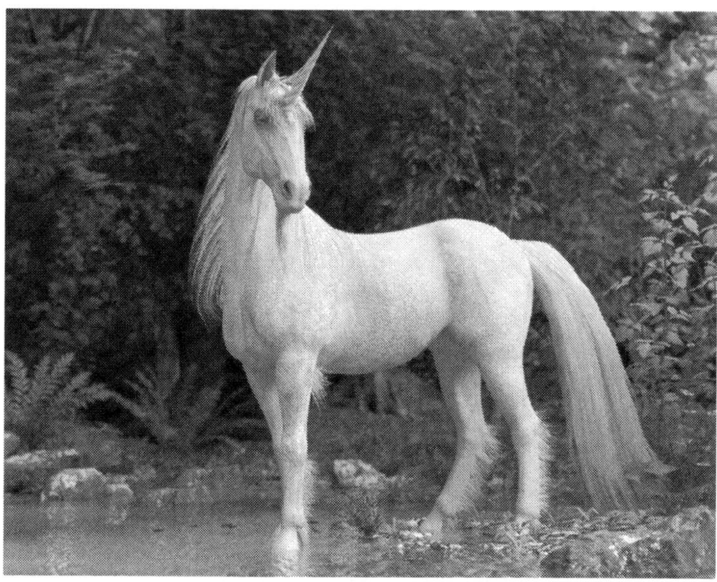

The perfect antibiotic is rarer than this.

After more than a century of research, you'd think we would have developed the perfect antibiotic. Unfortunately, this is not yet the case. The perfect antibiotic must meet a set of criteria, namely:

- It is toxic to the microbe but nontoxic to the host.
- It rapidly kills the pathogen outright rather than just slowly inhibiting further reproduction.
- It is delivered straight to the site of infection and functions even when diluted in body fluids.
- It remains potent until the infection is eliminated.
- It does not break down or exit the body before it has treated the infection.
- It works with the host's natural defenses to destroy all pathogenic bacteria, but ignores "good" bacteria in the gut and elsewhere.

- It has no major adverse reactions.
- It is unlikely to cause the body's immune system to react allergically.
- Its use does not lead to resistance on the part of the pathogen.
- It is reasonably priced and readily available.

As you can see, the above list sets a very high bar for any antibiotic. At present, there are antimicrobials that are effective against many diseases, but there is no cure-all drug that eliminates every infection. Penicillin, for example, kills many bacteria outright but its use (or, perhaps, overuse) has led to significant risk of resistance.

Other antibiotics have their own advantages and disadvantages. Every medicine has possible adverse reactions (side effects) such as diarrhea or stomach upset. Some of the newer antibiotics, while effective, are very costly.

Despite all their limitations, however, quite a few antibiotics fulfill their mission of killing the offending microbe, are reasonably priced, and generally well-tolerated by patients.

This is a good thing, but simply because you have an antibiotic on hand doesn't mean that particular one is good for all that ails you. Certain tools are needed for specific jobs. You wouldn't use a screwdriver to eat a steak or a steak knife to drive a screw into drywall; the same goes for antibiotics.

This doesn't mean that each antibiotic is only good against one type of bacteria; some, indeed, are best against a particular organism but many do double duty against different bugs.

Therefore, the effective medic must develop a fund of knowledge regarding different antibiotics. This involves more than simply knowing the dose of the medication and how many times a day you should take it. It's important to know how the drug works to eliminate an infection. The possible risks and available alternatives must also be understood to pinpoint the right therapy for the illness at hand.

EMPIRICAL VS. DEFINITIVE THERAPY

Every medical provider wants to be sure they are using the exact medicine needed to eliminate an infection. This is called the "**definitive therapy**. You have a reasonable certainty that it will cure the illness.

In austere settings without the benefit of lab studies, however, you are often basing your diagnosis purely on the patient's physical signs and symptoms.

You may be surprised to know that this is a very common way that physicians initiate treatment even with access to the most modern labs. When a caregiver suspects an infection, waiting for results to come back before starting treatment may not be in the patient's best interest.

Once you have made your educated guess, you choose an antibiotic likely to be successful in treating the illness. This is called "**empirical therapy**"; it is based on your experience in the absence of complete or perfect data.

A good analogy relates to hurricanes. There is a "cone of uncertainty" that shows possible tracks for a tropical cyclone in the near future. Meteorologists use their experience and knowledge of weather patterns to plot out this cone, but they aren't certain where landfall will occur. They are "empirically" making guesses as to where the storm will hit. Most of the time, they're correct.

We often mention diseases caused by a specific organism in this book. Unfortunately, you'll rarely have the good luck off the grid to know that an infection is caused by a specific bacterium, or that a certain antibiotic is guaranteed as a cure. By learning about different infections and antibiotics, you'll have the best chance to choose the correct "**empirical therapy**."

HOW ANTIBIOTICS WORK

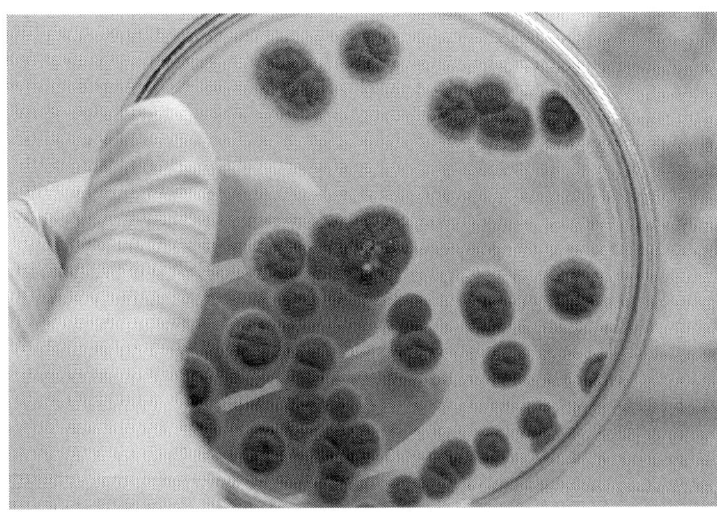

Penicillium fungus

It's common knowledge that there are medicines called antibiotics used for treating infection. Few people, however, know how antibiotics work to eliminate bacteria without doing damage to human cells. We know cancer chemotherapy may harm as well as help the patient, so how can something toxic to a bacterium not cause damage to the host it invades? By having its active effect target processes that exist only in the offending microbe.

Different organisms use different mechanisms to function. Bacteria reproduce, for example, by splitting in two, a process called binary fission. Humans reproduce by, well, other means. If antibiotics act on mechanisms that are unique to bacteria only, the infected host may experience no ill effect whatsoever.

Antibiotics work in two basic ways: By killing the infecting bacteria directly (a "**bactericidal**" effect), or by preventing repair and reproduction (a "**bacteriostatic**" effect). Some have the very useful quality of being effective against a wide range of bacteria. These drugs are known as "**broad**

spectrum" antibiotics. An example would be Fluoroquinolone drugs, which treat diseases like pneumonia, but are also often effective against urinary infections (and even anthrax!). Medications which target only a limited number or type of bacteria are called "**narrow spectrum**."

These bactericidal or bacteriostatic drugs work to eliminate infection in different ways. They may:

- Destroy or otherwise prevent access to substances required for bacteria to grow.
  Examples: Sulfa antibiotics (also called sulfonamides) target specific chemical reactions within a cell, blocking the ability of bacteria to use compounds that allow it to grow. Others, like erythromycin, bind to specific molecules that stop bacteria from forming the proteins they need to function.

- Prevent the mechanism by which bacteria repair damage to themselves.
  Examples: Levaquin is an antibiotic that stops bacterial overgrowth by preventing the repair of DNA genetic material. Other drugs that work in similar fashion include Ciprofloxacin (aka Cipro) and others.

- Destroy an essential part of the bacterium itself, like the cell wall.
  Examples: Penicillin works by disrupting the structure of the layer that keeps the bacteria intact (known as the cell "wall"). This kills it. Other antibiotics prevent certain bacteria from being able to build new walls.

- Inhibit reproduction so that the bacterial population dwindles and cannot sustain itself.
  Examples: Many Fluoroquinolones destroy the building blocks (lipids and proteins) that make up a cell's membrane and destroy DNA needed for bacterial multiplication. Rifamycin-type drugs, used to fight tuberculosis, inhibit the production of RNA, a "messenger" molecule

involved in passing information from the body's DNA needed to make essential proteins.

ANTIBIOTIC FAMILIES

Antibiotics with similar chemical makeup are categorized in groups sometimes referred to as "families." By grouping families according to their structure, we get antibiotics with common patterns of action as well as similar potential for toxicity. This allows us to have a general idea of what to expect when a particular antibiotic is used. Although drugs in an antibiotic family have some shared characteristics, each one is unique and must be studied individually.

Certain antibiotics, like penicillins and cephalosporins, are also designated by "generation." The first generation of these drugs were derived from natural products, with succeeding generations being, for the most part, synthetic. Each generation has different levels of activity against different organisms: earlier generations may be narrow-spectrum, for example, while later generations may be effective against a broader range of pathogens.

Some main classifications (individual antibiotics will be discussed later) include:

- Beta-Lactams
- Macrolides
- Fluoroquinolones
- Sulfonamides
- Tetracyclines
- Lincosamides
- Aminoglycosides
- Nitroimidazoles
- Rifamycins

Beta-Lactam Antibiotics (Penicillins And Others)

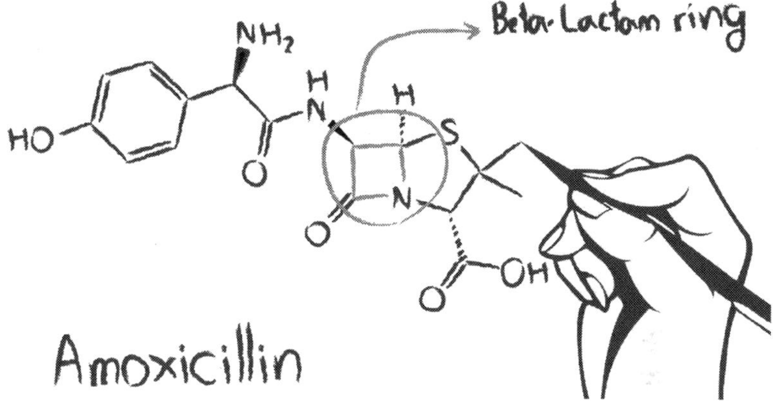

Beta-lactams are a class of generally broad-spectrum antibiotics that all contain a specific chemical structure called a "**beta-lactam ring**." This family includes penicillin, cephalosporins, and a number of other popular drugs, making them the most commonly used antibiotics. The position of the beta-lactam ring on the antibiotic molecule differentiates the various members of the family.

Beta lactam antibiotics target the outer surface of the cell (called a "membrane"). The beta-lactam ring of this group of antibiotics binds itself to certain bacterial proteins, rendering them unable to perform their role in producing strong cell walls. Specifically, they inhibit the production of **peptidoglycan**, a major component of the cell wall of Gram-positive bacteria. The resulting "leaky" cell walls are unstable and fall apart, leading to the death of the bacterium (a "bactericidal effect")

As one of the earliest and most frequently used antibiotics, Beta-Lactams have lost some of their effectiveness due to bacteria that have developed significant **resistance** against them. Microbes accomplish this feat by making a chemical called "beta-lactamase" that attacks the beta-lactam ring of penicillins and cephalosporins.

In response, some antibiotics in this family are now used in combination with drugs like clavulanic acid and sulbactam that inhibit the production of beta-lactamase, thus overcoming the bacteria's resistance. Although many antibiotics in this family have fallen victim to resistance issues, the Beta lactam known as "carbapenem" has been used as a drug of last resort in certain stubborn hospital-based infections.

Besides penicillins, a second groups of Beta-lactams include the Cephalosporins. Cephalexin (Keflex) is the most well-known of this group. These drugs are also in wide-spread use, with later generations often reserved to treat or prevent hospital-based or surgery-related infections. Of all the Beta-Lactams, amoxicillin, ampicillin, penicillin, and cephalexin are described in this book, as they all have veterinary equivalents available to the average citizen for storage purposes.

Aminoglycosides

Aminoglycosides are a family of antibacterial agents that inhibit protein synthesis in Gram-negative pathogens. They are so named because they contain an amino-modified glycoside (a type of sugar) in their chemical structure.

Streptomycin is an early aminoglycoside antibiotic that was the earliest modern agent used against tuberculosis. Tobramycin, gentamicin, and neomycin, all in common use today, were developed later.

Aminoglycosides have bactericidal action against most gram-negative **aerobic** and some **anaerobic** bacilli; they are less effective against the Gram-positive bacteria that Penicillin handles well. One advantage of aminoglycosides is that they act quickly to inhibit protein synthesis; thus, they are most effective against rapidly-multiplying bacterial populations.

Drugs in this family, however, are associated with various toxic effects, especially relating to hearing as well as kidney and liver function. They also are not options in most cases during pregnancy.

From the standpoint of use in disaster or other off-grid settings, these drugs are mostly given IV and have no veterinary equivalent, so access is very limited. It may surprise you to know that normal saline and other intravenous fluids are by prescription only; obtaining any meaningful quantity is problematic.

Lincosamides

Lincosamides prevent bacterial multiplication by interfering with the synthesis of proteins. They do this by blocking the transfer of genetic material from a tiny structure known as a "ribosome" in the cell. Ribosomes function as the site of protein manufacture and any obstacle to their function is ultimately fatal to the microbe. This does not usually kill the bacteria outright, but affects its function and reproduction to eventually eliminate the population. Antibiotics in this class are usually, therefore, considered to be bacteriostatic. At higher dosages, some drugs in this family can be bactericidal.

The lincosamides. Including clindamycin, lincomycin, and others. They show a reasonable broad-spectrum affect, especially against organisms that do not require oxygen to live (known as "**anaerobes**").

Anaerobic bacteria are more likely to exist in deep puncture wounds where the break in the skin is small. In these cases, less oxygen from the atmosphere can reach the bacteria, favoring **colonization** with anaerobes.

Lincosamides are rapidly absorbed and easily distribute into most tissues and body fluids, except perhaps for spinal fluid. A number are used to treat bone and joint infections, wound infections including MRSA, abscesses, oral infection, and some respiratory infections. They have a risk, however, of intestinal or liver toxicity and should be avoided in those with these medical issues. Clindamycin is discussed later in this book.

Macrolides

Antibiotics in the macrolide family are used to treat infections caused by gram-positive bacteria like *Streptococcus pneumoniae*. They are also generally effective against a limited range of gram-negative bacteria (e.g., *Haemophilus influenzae*), and some other causes of respiratory tract and soft-tissue infections.

Macrolides inhibit the synthesis of proteins needed for ribosomes to decode genetic material for reproduction. This action is considered to be bacteriostatic. Popular macrolides include erythromycin, azithromycin, and clarithromycin.

Macrolides are effective against a number of pathogens usually treated with penicillin-family drugs, such as beta-hemolytic streptococci, pneumococci, staphylococci, and enterococci. Therefore, they are often used as a substitute in those allergic to beta-lactam drugs.

Macrolides have also been shown to be effective against *Legionella pneumophila*, mycoplasmas, mycobacteria, some rickettsia, and *Chlamydia trachomatis*. In addition, some macrolides, like Amphotericin B and the popular drug nystatin, have antifungal action and are known as "**antimycotics**."

Like Lincosamides, some macrolides exhibit signs of liver and GI toxicity. Azithromycin and erythromycin will be discussed later in this book.

Sulfonamides

Sulfonamides, also known as "sulfa drugs," are one of the first antibiotics. They were commercially available even before penicillin and, as mentioned earlier, many WWII medic kits came with Sulfa powder to prevent infection.

Sulfa drugs eliminate infection by disabling processes required to make vital substances needed for bacterial **metabolism**. Sulfonamide compounds mimic a chemical called para-aminobenzoic acid or "PABA." PABA is needed for making a vitamin (B9) called folic acid. All cells need this vitamin and, although it easily enters human cells, it cannot enter bacterial cells. The bacteria are forced to manufacture it; Sulfonamides inhibit a critical chemical needed for this process. If folic acid cannot be made, bacteria stop growing. As the bacteria are not killed outright, sulfonamides are considered bacteriostatic.

Sulfa drugs are most well-known for their success in treating urinary infections in their brand name versions "Septra" or "Bactrim." This drug is actually a combination of two sulfonamides, sulfamethoxazole and Trimethoprim. In Great Britain, it may be recognized by the name co-trimoxazole.

The main side effects and adverse reactions are allergies and toxicity in the blood and kidneys. In rat studies, the use of this drug was seen to cause birth defects; therefore, it is not used during pregnancy. One negative to this otherwise useful medication is that sulfamethoxazole 400mg/Trimethoprim 80mg (referred to as SMZ/TMP) is well known to cause allergic reactions in some individuals. These reactions to sulfa drugs are almost as common as Penicillin allergies. We'll discuss this antibiotic in more detail later in the book.

Nitroimidazoles

The nitroimidazole family includes a number of bacteria that are known for their action against anaerobic bacteria as well as protozoa. Metronidazole is a commonly used member of this family.

The toxic effect of this family of antibiotics depends on a number of factors. They work by reducing part of the chemical structure of the offending microbe known as a "nitro" group. This allows the drug to more easily enter the cell. Once there, it facilitates the breakage of genetic material. It may also inhibit a bacteria's ability to repair the breakage.

Metronidazole is useful for the treatment of various infections with bacteria or protozoa that cause diarrheal diseases. Infection with these pathogens is usually as a result of water and food contamination. The main side effects are also related to the gastrointestinal tract. Metronidazole, also known as Flagyl, will be discussed later in this book.

Tetracyclines

Tetracyclines is one of the oldest antibiotic families, but a number of drugs in this group are important even today. Bacteriostatic in nature, these drugs prevent reproduction of offending organisms by inhibiting the manufacture of bacterial proteins.

Popular antibiotics in this class include doxycycline and minocycline. They are useful in genital infections, epidemic diseases like cholera and typhus, plus a number of respiratory infections.

The original tetracyclines were implicated in serious kidney ailments, especially if used when expired. Most of these reports were from decades ago, when the formulation for the drug was different than it is currently. The same experience doesn't seem to occur as often with later tetracyclines like doxycycline. Indeed, the government issued an emergency use authorization for expired doxycycline when a shortage of the drug hit the news several years ago.

Doxycycline is marketed under various names, including Vibramycin and Vibra-Tabs; its veterinary equivalent sometimes comes in powder packets. Doxycycline and minocycline will all be discussed later in this book.

Quinolones/Fluoroquinolones

Quinolones exert their bactericidal effect by interfering with a bacterium's ability to make DNA. This is accomplished by destroying certain chemicals essential for genetic replication.

Although still used for the treatment of malaria, early quinolones gave way to the next generation called "fluoroquinolones." These are more readily absorbed and more potent against gram-negative bacteria. The newer drugs are more broad-spectrum as well. Common fluoroquinolones in use today include Ciprofloxacin, ofloxacin, norfloxacin, and others.

Ciprofloxacin is an example of an antibiotic that has significant risks as well as benefits. Among a number of side effects, Cipro has been reported to cause weakness in muscles and tendons, and may negatively impact hearing. It may also cause joint issues in children. Therefore, it is restricted in pediatric use to only a very few infections. As well, Ciprofloxacin has not been deemed safe for use during pregnancy.

It is, however, one of those antibiotics acceptable for those allergic to penicillin. Ciprofloxacin will be described later in this book.

Rifamycins/Ansamycins

Rifamycins are a subgroup of the ansamycin family originally developed from *Streptomyces* bacteria, but also synthetically manufactured today. Rifamycins inhibit the production of RNA genetic material in the bacterial cell.

The rifamycin family is especially valuable to combat infections with bacteria in the *mycobacteria* class. Mycobacteria are the causes of tuberculosis, leprosy, and a number of other major infections.

I have personal experience with mycobacteria. During my residency, I worked in inner-city emergency rooms in Miami during the 1980 Mariel boatlift. Due to relatively lax isolation standards in that time period, I converted to positive for tuberculosis and had to take six months of combination therapy with rifamycins and other drugs. Even today, I carry x-ray evidence of the now-dormant infection.

Unfortunately, rifamycins are toxic to the GI tract and liver, subject to a number of restrictions, and not available in veterinary equivalents.

Other antibiotic families exist, but none that are available to the average citizen for long-term disaster storage.

SIDE EFFECTS VS. ALLERGIES

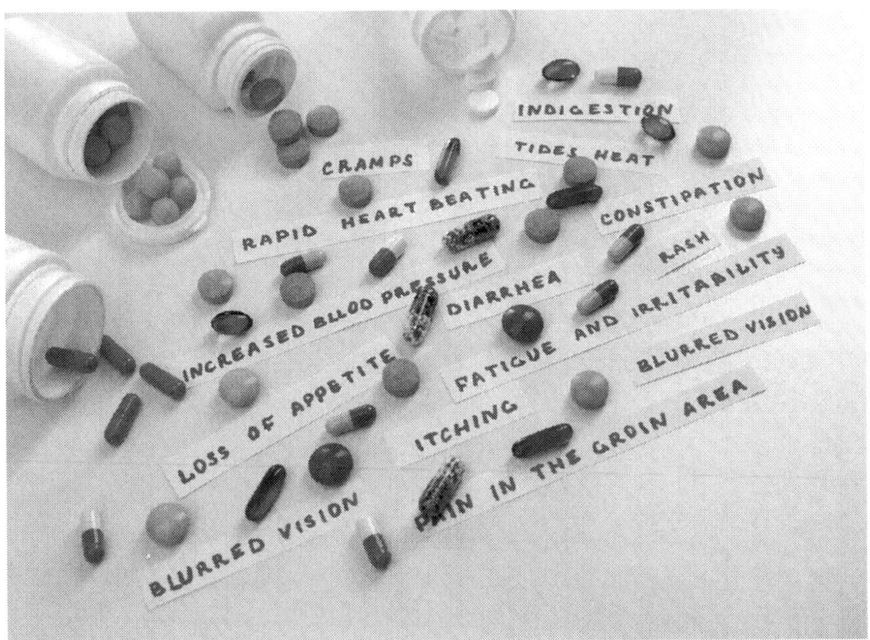

Although an antibiotic might cure an infection, it is not without its risks. In addition to its primary beneficial effect, the chemical compounds in the drug may have **"side" effects**. No medicine is without the risk of an adverse reaction.

Adverse reactions may be different from a medication **allergy**, although both are relatively common occurrences. When deciding whether to use a medicine, a caregiver must always ask the patient if they have had any negative experience with it or a similar medicine.

The response they receive may be unclear, however, as to whether an allergy exists or the patient simply had a known side effect.

Many people will report that they are allergic to a particular drug. The reasons for this could be:

- It caused symptoms that made them feel unwell.
- A family member was once diagnosed as being allergic to the drug and they assume they might be also.
- Their parents told them about an incident during childhood that resembled an allergy, so better safe than sorry.
- They read something negative about the drug in the media or online and they don't want to take it.
- They are philosophically opposed to a particular type of drug, such as psychotropics.
- They might actually be allergic to the drug.

We place a true allergy to a drug last on this list because, according to the World Allergy Organization, less than 10% of reactions to medications actually relate to allergies. Indeed, most negative effects that people experience after taking medicine are simply adverse reactions.

How can you tell the difference and why does it matter? A **drug allergy** is a negative response by your immune system after exposure to a medicine. A "**side-effect**," on the other hand, is a negative consequence of its use *expected* to occur in a (hopefully) small percentage of patients. Side-effects are well-documented in research studies when the drug is developed or in reports from patients after it is released on the open market.

For example: If a drug is well-known to cause, say, abdominal cramps in a percentage of people, then abdominal cramps would be a side-effect instead of an allergy. If a medicine causes, instead, an immune response, such as the rapid onset of rashes, swelling, and difficulty breathing, it is more likely an allergy. If inability to breathe were a known side effect of a drug, it's unlikely that it would be made available to the general public. Having said this, some allergy-like effects are sometimes called "side effects."

Antibiotic Allergies

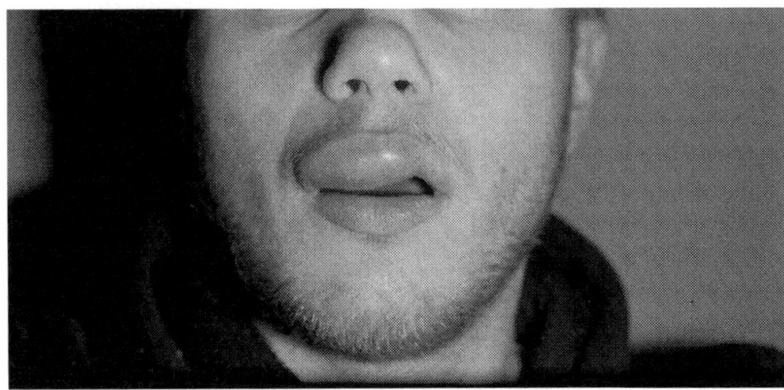

Allergic reaction affecting lip

In an allergic reaction, your immune system recognizes a substance as foreign. That's its job and it's pretty darn good at it. Once the immune system identifies an invader, it begins a cascade of actions that is normally protective. When that process goes haywire, however, it may become very harmful.

Usually, the immune system will not over-react the first time it's exposed to a drug. In order to respond "allergically," the body normally needs to be primed to the allergy-causing substance (also known as an "**allergen**"). We have heard of people claiming an allergic response the "first" time they take a medicine; We believe, however, that this occurred, if a true allergy, due to an unknown or inadvertent previous exposure. Allergies to many substances, including some drugs, can be determined by skin or blood tests.

Why is it important to know whether a symptom is related to a side effect or an allergy?

Here's an example: A man has chest pain and a history of heart disease. You suspect a heart attack, but he says that he is allergic to aspirin, the only medicine you have available on a backcountry camping trip. Do you give it?

Here's another: A woman has a severe infection that has proven resistant to many antibiotics, leaving you, the medic in a remote setting, with only one or two options. Both are listed as allergies in her medical history. What do you do?

Despite the apparent history of allergies to the medication in the two cases above, you may have to choose to give the drug to save the patient. Unfortunately, it may be deadly if they are truly allergic, so it is important to ask exactly what happened when the alleged allergic reaction occurred.

To confuse a side effect as an allergy ties a medical provider's hands and can cause a big difference in the final outcome. In austere settings where the choice of drugs is extremely limited, the caregiver becomes less effective if they can't use all the tools and supplies at their disposal.

Antibiotic Side Effects

The list of antibiotic side effects is too long to list in a book this length, but they commonly include skin inflammation leading to rashes and stomach upset with diarrhea. These adverse reactions are usually mild, but can be severe enough to merit avoiding or discontinuing the drug. In some rarer circumstances, adverse effects may be very dangerous, affecting the kidneys, liver, or other organs. Some common risks for selected antibiotics are discussed later in this book.

One adverse reaction seen with the use of many antibiotics is the fungal, or "yeast," infection. Antibiotics are well-known to cause overgrowths of yeast, especially in the vagina and oral cavity. These infections are usually associated with itching or burning and can cause significant irritation.

Fungal infections occur in these circumstances due to the fact that many antibiotics kill both the bacteria causing the infection and good bacteria that naturally inhabit your body.

Ordinarily, the good bacteria in these areas keep fungal organisms under control. Once an antibiotic has cleared the neighborhood, the balance has been disrupted; non-bacterial organisms like yeast may multiply opportunistically. Anti-fungal medications like Lotrimin (clotrimazole) or Diflucan (fluconazole) may be needed to control this growth until good bacteria are able to repopulate the area.

SELECTING AN ANTIBIOTIC

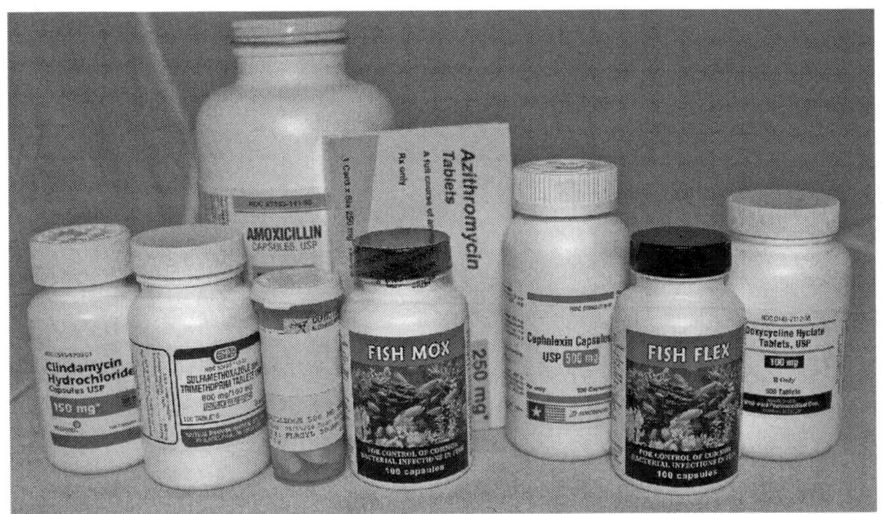

The decision to use antibiotics shouldn't be taken lightly, but when it is clear that an antibiotic is necessary, simply throwing a random drug at the patient is not the answer. Certain antibiotics are effective against some microbes, but may not eliminate others.

The opposite may also be true in particular cases. Different antibiotics may be used for the same condition, based on the offending organism, history of allergies, and other issues. As well, more than one antibiotic may be necessary to eliminate a stubborn or severe infection.

Some antibiotics may be more effective given in a certain way. For example, an antibiotic cream may be more appropriate for a skin infection than the same medicine taken in oral form. In other instances, an antibiotic may have to be administered intravenously to be successful in treating widespread infections such as **sepsis**.

Factors that must be taken into consideration include:

- The identity of the disease-causing organism
- The site of the infection
- The general health of the infected person
- The level of resistance of the specific organism to the antibiotics available

All of the above may be difficult to identify in austere settings. Without lab studies, it may be very unlikely you'll know exactly which organism caused the infection. Notable exceptions might include tetanus, which has a distinct presentation that's hard to miss (discussed earlier). It would probably be impossible to predict if the microbe is resistant or not to the usual antibiotic therapy.

You will have to make assumptions about the general health of the sick individual. A person may look healthy but could have heart or kidney problems possibly impacted by the antibiotic. The site of infection if often obvious, as with a skin abscess, but less so if internal organs are involved.

All of which makes your job complex in situations where the miracle of modern medicine is not at your fingertips. This doesn't signify that you have no chance of identifying the infection and treating it correctly. It means you are employing **empirical therapy** based on your experience, knowledge, and perhaps, some educated guesses.

STOCKPILING MEDICATIONS

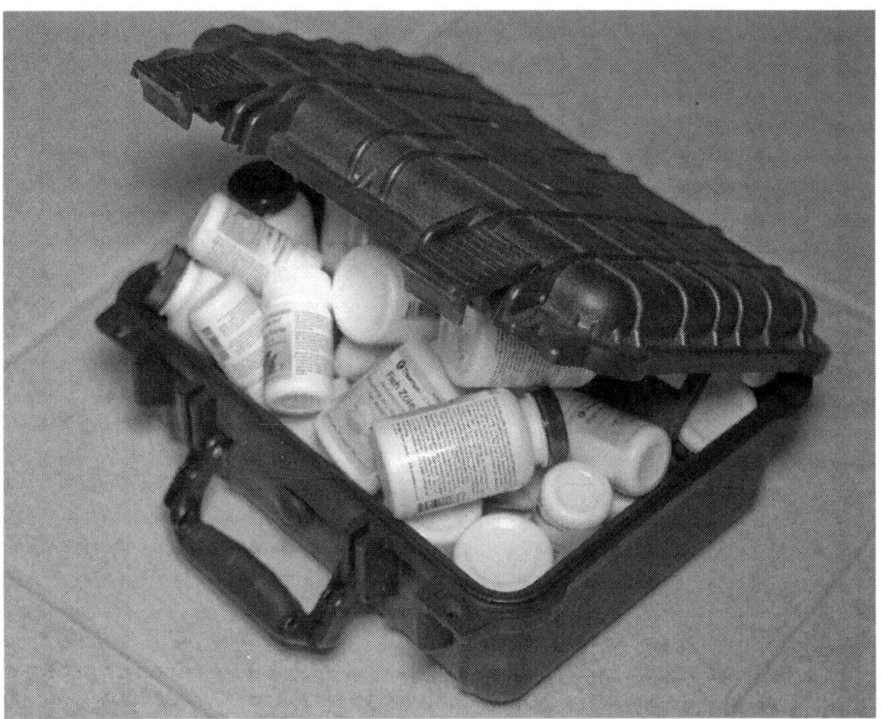

Accumulating over-the-counter drugs for the off-grid medicine cabinet may be simple. Obtaining antibiotics, however, is another matter altogether.

Unless you actually have an infection, most physicians wouldn't accommodate a request for these medications. This reluctance is not only to prevent allegations of malpractice, but also to combat the epidemic of antibiotic resistance in recent times. Even a sympathetic provider would balk at providing more than one course of treatment, not nearly enough to cover a family's long-term needs.

Yet, antibiotics are a class of medications that would be very useful, even life-saving, in austere scenarios. On a remote homestead or in an underdeveloped country, the inability to obtain these drugs may cost lives. This hard reality complicates the ability of a medic to be effective in the aftermath of a long-term disaster.

In any major catastrophe, there will be a much larger incidence of infection, not only from injuries and illness but from activities of daily survival. People who have to fend for themselves perform duties to which they're not accustomed. We don't know about you, but we haven't chopped wood for fuel much lately.

Any break in the skin leaves the body prone to infection. Within a short period of time, redness, swelling, and other signs of bacterial invasion will appear.

Treatment of such infections at an early stage improves the chance they will heal quickly and completely. Antibiotics are an integral part of that treatment; their availability would allow the possibility of dealing with the issue before it becomes life-threatening.

Without them, we are thrown back to the 19th century from a medical standpoint. It was a time when many rugged individualists "toughed it out," at least until their infection spread throughout their bodies. You can guess the probable end result.

Talking To Your Doctor

It's clear that antibiotics would be useful to have in your medical kit in tough times, but these are prescription drugs. Of course, a small quantity can be obtained by anyone who tells their doctor that they are leaving the country and would like to avoid "Travelers' Diarrhea." If you discuss your concerns about getting sick at the beginning of flu season, you'll probably get a prescription for the anti-viral drug Tamiflu.

This is all well and good for one or two courses of therapy, but a long-term alternative is required for the "medic" to have enough antibiotics to protect a family.

You might begin by having a serious and honest discussion with a healthcare provider. It should be someone with whom you have a long-standing relationship. Describe your concerns about not having needed medications in a disaster situation.

You don't have to describe the disaster as a complete societal collapse or zombie apocalypse. This will make you appear like the camouflage-wearing, gun-toting survivalists on reality shows. These programs have given the public, and perhaps your doctor, the wrong idea about people interested in preparedness; folks who, for the most part, are perfectly normal but serious about being ready to deal with disasters.

Truly, any catastrophe could leave you without access to your doctor for an extended period. It's only common sense to have a plan of action for situations where you can't reach them. A letter at the end of this book may help if given to your local physician. A printer-friendly version can be found on our survival medicine website at www.doomandbloom.net.

AQUARIUM AND AVIAN ANTIBIOTICS

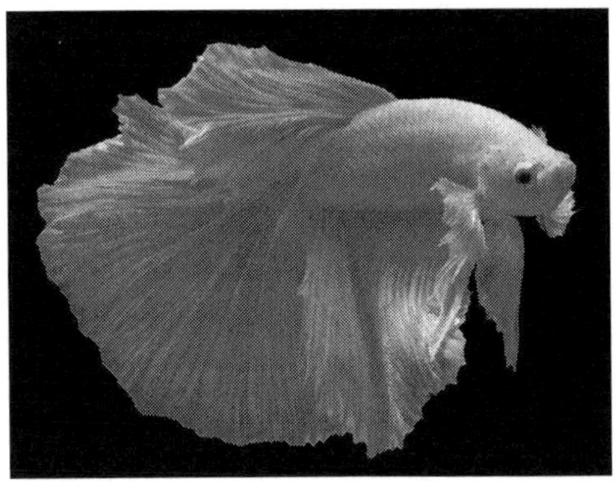

No matter how sympathetic your healthcare provider may be, it's unlikely that you'll be able to obtain a supply of antibiotics that would last for long if you're thrown off the grid. Injuries will occur as you perform activities to which you're not accustomed; injuries that can get infected. Even the water may be questionable, with pathogens that may cause infection as well.

As medical professionals, we hoped to find a way to decrease the number of infection-related deaths. There is a viable option: aquarium and avian antibiotics.

You may have had to re-read the last sentence to make sure you saw it correctly. Yes, we said aquarium and avian antibiotics. How can we possibly make such a statement?

The Case For "Fish Antibiotics"

For many years, we have had tropical fish in our home. When the times required us to become more self-sufficient, we set up a pond to raise tilapia. We also have a pet parrot that is now over 30 years old. It can be said that we know our way around fish and birds.

After decades of using aquatic medicines for fish and avian medicines for birds when needed, we decided to evaluate these drugs for their potential use in austere settings. It stood to reason that, without a functioning modern medical system, a strategy would be necessary for the average person to save a sick family member. Despite this, obtaining any significant amount of prescription antibiotics was problematic, to say the least.

Certain veterinary medicines seemed to be good candidates: All were widely available in different varieties, and didn't require a medical license to obtain them. In a long-term disaster scenario, having a supply of these could save lives. But should serious consideration be given to the idea of veterinary meds for use by humans, even those thrown off the grid for the foreseeable future? And would *any* pet drug be safe to take? At first, we looked at this proposition with skepticism.

A close inspection of the ingredients was in order to further our investigation. We evaluated the fish antibiotic known as Fish-Mox Forte. Reading the ingredients, this medication had exactly one: amoxicillin 500 mg, a common antibiotic used in humans. There were no additional chemicals added that made scales shinier or fins longer.

The dosage was also interesting: 500 milligrams is the dose of amoxicillin given to an adult human. As we researched further, we discovered that Fish-Mox *only* came in human dosages. Why does a guppy require the same amount of amoxicillin as a human? It was suggested that it's because you place it in the water, but there were no specific instructions we could find at the time that told us how much to add to the fish tank. Is one capsule the dose for a 100-gallon aquarium or is it the dose for a bowl?

Our question became: Is this medicine for fish identical to the amoxicillin made for human consumption? To determine this, only a direct comparison would do. We opened a bottle of amoxicillin 500 mg intended for humans (manufactured by DAVA Pharmaceuticals). We found red and pink capsules with the numbers and letters WC 731 on it. When we opened a bottle of Fish-Mox Forte, we found red and pink capsules with the numbers and letters WC 731 on it. The two were identical.

At first, we found it hard to believe, but discussions with a number of professionals in the pharmaceutical field confirmed our suspicions. The amoxicillin used in humans was also packaged and distributed as a medication for fish with bacterial infections.

Over time, we found about a dozen aquarium and avian antibiotics that met a very specific set of criteria:

- The veterinary drug must have only one ingredient, the antibiotic itself.
- The drug, although marketed for pets, must only be produced in dosages used in human adults or children.
- The veterinary drug and human version must be identical to each other down to the identification letters and numbers.
- The medication must be available without a prescription
- The medication must be available for purchase in bulk.

As you can imagine, very few antibiotic medications used in the veterinary field meet these criteria. Antibiotics for large animals like horses aren't produced in human dosages. Evaluation of many cat, dog, and livestock antibiotics often revealed additives that might cause ill effects on a human being.

Sometimes the extra ingredients are inert by-products of manufacturing that are too costly to remove just for use on animals. Regardless, we believe it is safer to look only for those veterinary drugs that have the antibiotic as the *sole* ingredient.

In our original version of this book, we listed the products that met our criteria at the time of writing. We believed (and still do) that having a supply of these would be useful additions to any medical kit, not just for major long-term disasters, but for use in remote homesteads, long backcountry expeditions, or medical missions to underdeveloped countries. They were:

- FISH-MOX (Amoxicillin 250 mg)
- FISH_MOX FORTE (Amoxicillin 500 mg)
- FISH-CILLIN (Ampicillin 250 mg)
- FISH-FLEX (Cephalexin 250 mg)
- FISH-FLEX FORTE (Cephalexin 500 mg)
- FISH-ZOLE (Metronidazole 250 mg)
- FISH-ZOLE FORTE (Metronidazole 500 mg)
- FISH-PEN (Penicillin 250 mg)
- FISH-PEN FORTE (Penicillin 500 mg)
- FISH-FLOX (Ciprofloxacin 250 mg)
- FISH-FLOX FORTE (Ciprofloxacin 500 mg)
- FISH-CIN (Clindamycin 150 mg)
- FISH-MIN (Minocycline 50 Or 100 mg)
- FISH-MYCIN (Erythromycin 250 mg)
- FISH-DOXY (Doxycycline 100 mg)
- BIRD-BIOTIC (Doxycycline 100 mg)
- BIRD-SULFA (Sulfamethoxazole 400 mg/Trimethoprim 80mg)
- FISH-SULFA FORTE (Sulfamethoxazole 800 mg/ Trimethoprim 160mg)
- BIRD-ZITHRO (Azithromycin 250 mg)
- FISH-FLUCON (Fluconazole 100 mg)

These medications were available without a prescription online. They usually came in lots of 12 to 100 capsules or powder packets, often for less than the retail price of the same prescription medication at the local pharmacy. Other brands exist today that are packaged the same way.

If you so desired, you could get as much as you can afford to stockpile for use in a mission overseas or other austere setting. For those responsible for a large family or group, this aspect is perhaps one of the most important reasons to consider these products; such quantities would be impossible to obtain even from the most sympathetic physician.

Of course, anyone could be allergic to one or another of these antibiotics, but it would be a very rare individual who would be allergic to all of them. There is a possibility for **cross-reactivity** with regards to allergies: a 10% chance for cross-reactivity exists, for example, between penicillin drugs and cephalexin (Keflex). If you are allergic to penicillin, you could also be allergic to Keflex.

It would be hypocritical to suggest that a veterinary antibiotic is usable in humans without testimony. Here's ours: We have personally used some (not all) of these antibiotics on our own persons without any ill effects. Whenever we have used them, the results have been indistinguishable from human antibiotics, something you might expect since they are, indeed, the same medication, identical in appearance and dosage.

A Changing Landscape

It's interesting to see what has happened since we first wrote about veterinary antibiotics in austere scenarios. Fish antibiotic distributors now publish easy-to-find instructions that tell you how much to use depending on the size of the aquarium.

In response to outside pressure, some of these drugs were withdrawn from the pet market altogether. As a matter of fact, a brand known as Fish-Cycline, a veterinary version of tetracycline, was removed from the market as this book was being written. Since publication, all the antibiotic brands listed above have been withdrawn from the market. Luckily, many have been replaced by new brands of the same drug, but the market is volatile. Search for the generic antibiotic name and you'll find them.

To make the antibiotics appear different from the human versions, some of the above antibiotics now come in powder packets to make it seem like they're a different product.

It's important to remember that these medications are meant for situations where there is not a functioning modern medical system. We do not recommend self-treatment in any circumstance that does not involve the complete long-term loss of access to medical care. Let's face it, the practice of medicine without a license is illegal and punishable by law. They say that a person who acts as his own lawyer has a fool for a client; in normal times, leave it to the professionals.

Penicillin Allergy Alternatives

Those who can't take penicillin have suitable safe alternatives in the group of antibiotics mentioned in this book. Any of the antibiotics below should not cause a reaction in a patient allergic to penicillin-family drugs:

- Doxycycline
- Metronidazole
- Tetracycline
- Ciprofloxacin
- Levofloxacin
- Clindamycin
- Sulfa Drugs
- Azithromycin
- Minocycline

THE WISE USE OF ANTIBIOTICS

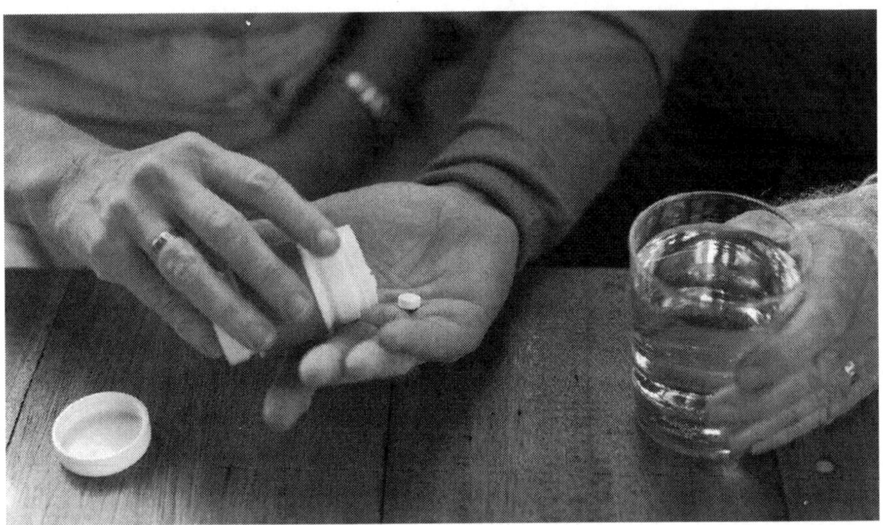

If antibiotics are treated like candy, their overuse will cause even more issues with bacterial resistance than we have now. The wise use of these medications involves developing a fund of knowledge for each one.

Although you might think that any antibiotic will work to cure any disease, this is not the case. Specific antibiotics should be used at specific doses for specific illnesses. The exact dosage of each and every antibiotic for every disease in existence is, however, beyond the scope of a book this size. Although we mention some common side effects of the antibiotics we discuss, rare effects could number in the dozens for each drug.

Despite this book's limitations, it's important to have as much information as possible on medications that you plan to obtain and store. This information is available in many places, such as the Merck Manual or the Physician's Desk Reference, popularly known as "The PDR." The PDR is available in digital or app form, and has just about every bit of information that exists on a particular drug, including photos. Older editions of the PDR exist in printed version, and are still useful except for the very latest drugs. They can be found on places like online auction sites. Other online sources are good options: As of this writing, sites like drugs.com or rxlist.com have the information you need.

The book you're reading has a very specific purpose: To provide information about antibiotics that come in veterinary equivalents without a prescription. The PDR, Merck Manual, and other sources can give you even more extensive details about prescription medications, down to the very rarest side effect.

Using these resources will provide a huge amount of information. Under each and every medicine currently on the market, you will find every "**indication**" (the medical conditions that the drug is used for). Also listed will be every dosage for every disease, every possible risk or interaction, and numerous side effects.

ANTIBIOTIC RESISTANCE

HOW ANTIBIOTIC RESISTANCE HAPPENS

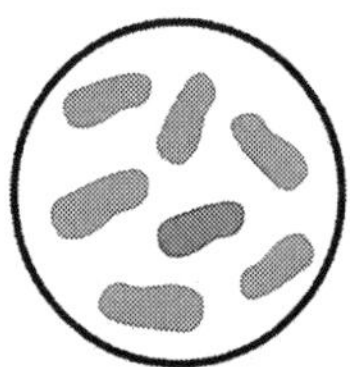

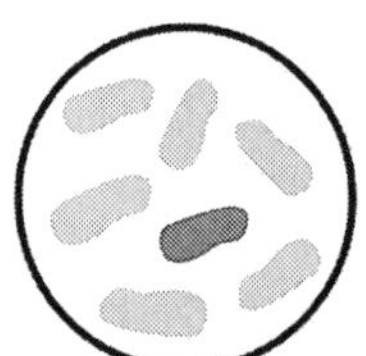

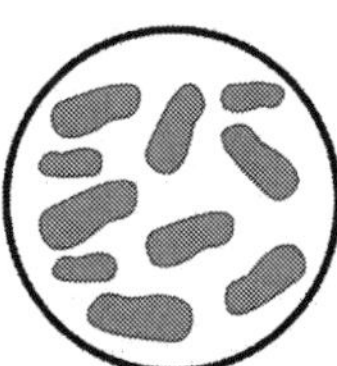

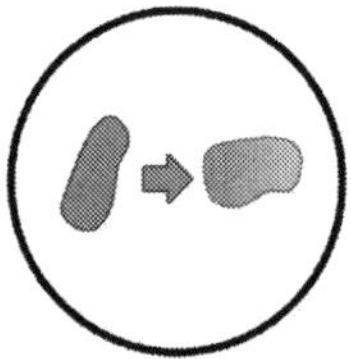

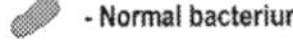

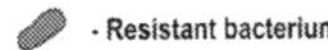

When modern medical care isn't available, many deaths would be prevented by the availability of antibiotics in your disaster medicine cabinet. Indeed, you should consider having a supply of these drugs in your storage if you believe a disaster may occur that takes away your access to modern medical care.

If you use antibiotics for every minor ailment that comes along, however, you will run out very quickly and may contribute to an epidemic of **antibiotic resistance** caused by overuse.

Resistant organisms develop ways to deactivate or otherwise circumvent an antibiotic's action. In the case of penicillin resistance, some bacteria began to produce a chemical that broke down the beta-lactam ring in the structure of penicillin family drugs (also called "beta-lactams"). This chemical, known as beta-lactamase, rendered the antibiotic ineffective.

Antibiotics are essential tools for success in long-term survival. Unfortunately, the government, the livestock industry, and some physicians have fostered widespread resistance to many of the standard drugs. Even patients themselves put pressure on their health providers for antibiotic prescriptions. The Centers for Disease Control and Prevention report that a significant percentage of people leave their doctor's office with an antibiotic prescription that is of absolutely no use to treat their *viral* infection (or no infection at all)!

Make no mistake, antibiotic overuse is an epidemic: More than 2 million diagnosed cases of antibiotic resistance were reported in the United States in 2013, leading to 23,000 deaths and costing 30 billion dollars.

As of 2015, The Center for Disease Control and Prevention had compiled a list of close to 20 bacteria that have shown a tendency towards antibiotic resistance. They include various organisms that cause severe diarrheal disease, respiratory issues, wound infections, and even sexually transmitted disease.

The CDC's list:

- *Clostridium difficile*
- Carbapenem-resistant *Enterobacteriaceae* (CRE)
- Drug-resistant *Neisseria gonorrhoeae*
- Multidrug-resistant *Acinetobacter*
- Drug-resistant *Campylobacter*
- Fluconazole-resistant *Candida*
- Extended spectrum β-lactamase producing *Enterobacteriaceae* (ESBLs)
- Vancomycin-resistant *Enterococcus* (VRE)
- Multidrug-resistant *Pseudomonas aeruginosa*
- Drug-resistant Non-typhoidal *Salmonella*
- Drug-resistant *Salmonella typhi*
- Drug-resistant *Shigella*
- Methicillin-resistant *Staphylococcus aureus* (MRSA)
- Drug-resistant *Streptococcus pneumoniae*
- Multidrug-resistant *mycobacteria tuberculosis*
- Vancomycin-resistant *Staphylococcus aureus* (VRSA)
- Erythromycin-resistant Group A *Streptococcus*
- Clindamycin-resistant Group B *Streptococcus*

There have been no effective treatments identified for some of the above microbes, as in the case of multidrug-resistant Tuberculosis. Methicillin-Resistant Staph. aureus (MRSA) has been responsible for more deaths than AIDS in recent years.

Even when prescribed appropriately by the physician, the actions of some patients contribute to the resistance epidemic. Many times, people will feel better after taking the first two or three days of a seven to ten-day course of an antibiotic. They then stop, assuming the infection has been eliminated.

Indeed, most of the bacteria are dead, but some colonies may persist if you prematurely end the treatment. A stubborn one percent multiplies and becomes the vanguard for a stronger, more resistant infection.

We understand that, in a long-term scenario, you may be tempted to use an antibiotic for a shorter time to conserve your last few pills. In a true long-term disaster, where no chance of obtaining replacement medicine exists, it may leave you with some tough decisions. Just be aware that the best way of eliminating an infection is completing the full course of treatment.

Those entrusted with the health of family members after a disaster must serve as the medical quartermaster. Wisely dispensing the medications available will not only save lives but also conserve the precious and scarce supply that would be all you have if some major event occurs. You must walk a fine line between observant patient management (doing nothing) and aggressive management (doing everything).

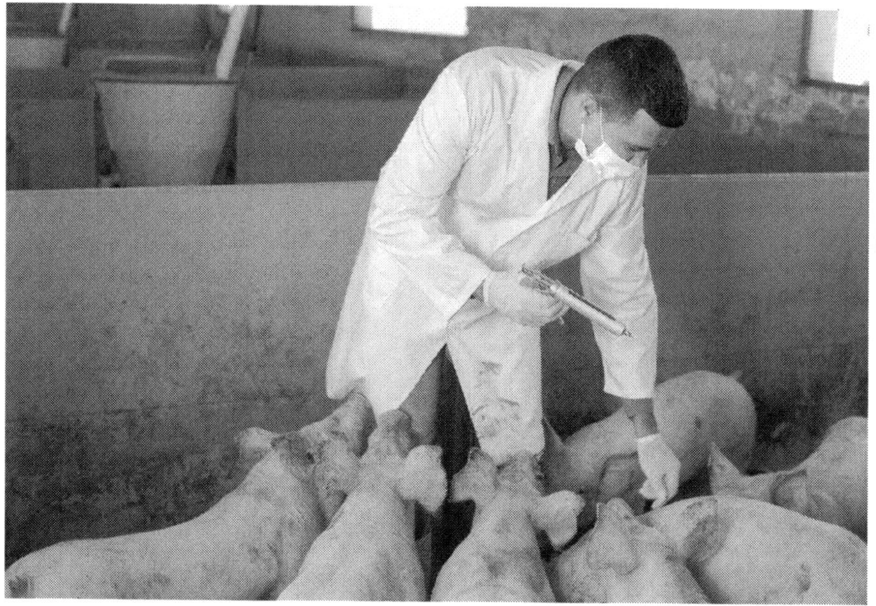

Most antibiotics go to food-producing livestock, not humans

The liberal use of antibiotics is a poor strategy for a few reasons:

- Overuse can foster the spread of resistant bacteria. In the 2011 salmonella outbreak, millions of pounds of antibiotic-laden turkey meat were discarded after 100 people were sent to the hospital with severe diarrheal disease. The food industry is responsible for 80% of the antibiotic use in the U.S. This is not used to treat sick livestock, but to make healthy livestock grow faster and get to market sooner. Routine use of antibiotics on food-producing animals is not required nor is it beneficial. Some European countries, like Denmark, forbid the routine use of antibiotics in livestock without any apparent detriment to public health. Consider supporting farmers who raise antibiotic-free livestock; this will decrease the further development of resistant bacteria, and, thus, the antibiotics you have will be more effective.

- Potential allergic reactions may occur that could lead to **anaphylactic shock**. Frequent exposure to antibiotics increases the likelihood of developing an allergy to one or more of them.
- Many infections, including most respiratory infections, are viral; antibiotics are completely ineffective in treating them. The common cold, for example, is a viral illness. Antibiotics would be no more effective to eliminate it than breath mints.
- Lastly, being trigger-happy with antibiotics may make diagnosing an illness more difficult. If you give antibiotics before you're sure what medical problem you're actually dealing with, you might "mask" the condition. In other words, symptoms that could help figure out what disease your patient has might temporarily disappear. This costs you valuable time in determining the correct treatment.

Rehydration, rest, and symptomatic relief (for example, ibuprofen to relieve fever) may be the most appropriate first course of action for most infections. The body may eliminate the bacteria and its toxins on its own, so consider the use of these drugs only for serious disease. The logic behind this recommendation is twofold:

1) Antibiotics have side-effects. You might give a drug for, say, an infectious diarrhea only to find that its main side effect is...diarrhea.
2) Unless you own a pharmaceutical company, you'll have only a limited supply of medicine. In a disaster, replacing those drugs will be difficult or impossible, so you'll want to use them only when absolutely necessary.

It should be noted that that the director of the CDC (Centers for Disease Control) has advocated an increased "stewardship" of veterinary antibiotics due to the epidemic of antibiotic resistance. Vigilance is required, and rightly so, to stop the epidemic of antibiotic resistance we're seeing today. As a result, we can expect access to antibiotics to be curtailed even more in the future.

In January 2018, the government chose to eliminate availability of a number of veterinary antibiotics to the general public. This initiative was called the Veterinary Feed Directive, and ended access to a wide range of antibiotics unless prescribed by a veterinarian.

Fortunately, the antibiotic options mentioned in this book are made for the ornamental or pet industry and not for, as the Veterinary Feed Directive implies, food-producing livestock. None of these meds are used in any large-scale operation meant to bring food to the table.

This doesn't mean that aquarium and avian antibiotics might not, one day, be removed from the market, at least without a veterinarian's prescription. Whether this is something that is likely to happen is uncertain; how many people bring sick guppies or goldfish to veterinarians? Despite this, the wise individual who is concerned about the loss of modern medical care in a disaster might consider obtaining a supply for their "austere medicine cabinet" sooner than later.

The judicious use of antibiotics under close supervision is required to utilize their benefits without increasing their risks. In austere settings where modern care is unavailable, it will be tempting to use up whatever supply of antibiotics exist. Discourage family members from taking these drugs without first consulting the person medically responsible for the family's or group's health. In normal times, of course, seek the advice of a qualified medical professional.

ANTIFUNGAL AND ANTIVIRAL DRUGS

This book is specifically about antibiotics, which are most effective against bacteria and protozoa. Antibiotics will not cure the common cold, herpes, Ebola, or any other disease caused by a virus.

Antibiotics don't affect a viral infection one way or another, but the use of antibiotics actually causes fungal infections by eliminating good bacteria as well as bad from the body, leaving lots of room for opportunistic fungal organisms to take over.

This doesn't mean that it is unreasonable to have a supply of Tamiflu (Oseltamivir) in advance of flu season. Influenza is still a major cause of deaths, especially among the elderly. Tamiflu, although not very effective for a lot of other viruses, is most useful for the flu if used within 48 hours of the start of symptoms. The FDA has approved Tamiflu for use in everyone 2 weeks of age or older.

From an anti-fungal standpoint, fluconazole is a popular medication useful to treat or prevent a variety of yeast infections. It will be described in more detail later in this book.

NATURAL ANTIBIOTICS

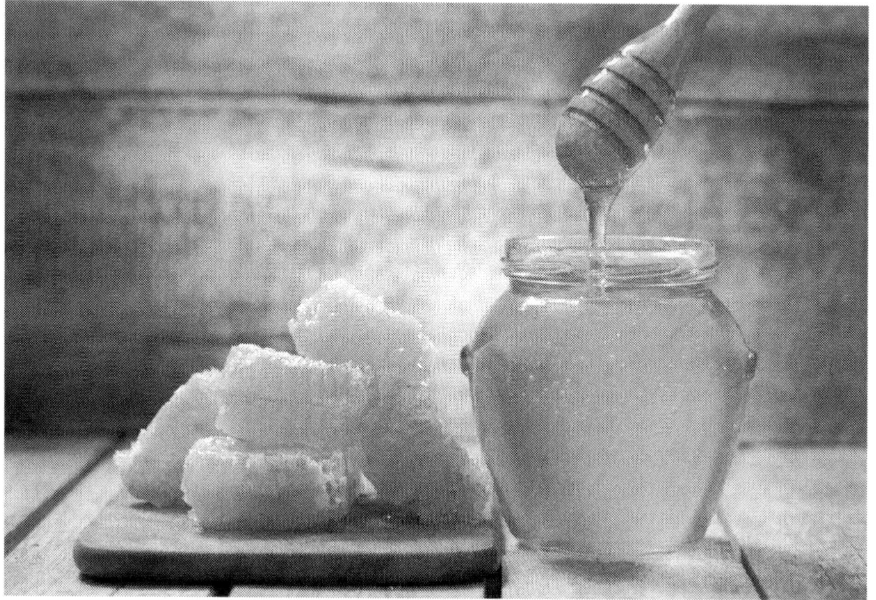

Raw unprocessed honey is a natural antibiotic

A number of natural substances have been described as effective in the treatment of infection. These include products like raw unprocessed honey, onion, and garlic. A discussion of these is a topic so complex that it requires its own volume.

Suffice it to say that anyone concerned about a long-term disaster throwing them off the grid should realize that, eventually, the supply of antibiotic drugs will run out. As a matter of fact, it will be likely that these medicines will be expended quickly and will be difficult, if not impossible, to replace.

Given the likelihood that a major long-term disaster will eliminate most, if not all, modern medical options, it is simple logic that we should examine the strategies employed by previous generations to treat disease. If you look at medical books from the 19th century, you will see that herbal medicine, considered alternative healing now, was once standard conventional medicine.

A working medicinal garden is what our ancestors used to keep their families healthy. Starting your own would be a valuable addition to your backyard as well. Those interested in further study on herbal antibiotics might consider these reference guides:

- ***Herbal Antibiotics*** by Buhner
- ***The Encyclopedia of Herbal Medicine*** by Chevallier
- ***Medical Herbalism*** by Hoffman

Although this is not a book on herbal antibiotics, we would be remiss if we didn't mention the antibiotic properties of raw unprocessed honey. This is not the opinion of alternative healers, but, rather, the results of numerous studies performed by conventional scientists.

Honey is one of the oldest known antiseptic dressings; it was used by the ancient Greeks for infected wounds. The healing properties of honey are mentioned in the Bible, Koran, and Torah.

If we are ever thrown back medically to the 19th century due to some event, we will have to improvise medical strategies that we perhaps might be reluctant to consider today. Never ignore avenues that may help you gain access to more tools in the medical woodshed that can fight infectious diseases.

The chemicals in honey work to kill various bacterial and fungal species. Applied to the skin or open wounds, honey may serve as a barrier to moisture. It tends to keep skin from sticking to bandages, causing less pain during wound cleanings. Honey may also provide nutrients that speed wound healing.

Some reports describe the action of honey or honey-soaked dressings on different types of wounds, including surgical incisions, bedsores, abscesses, and burns. Evidence suggests that honey reduces pus and odor in wound infections and may even decrease the time to full recovery.

SECTION 4

+++

INDIVIDUAL ANTIBIOTICS

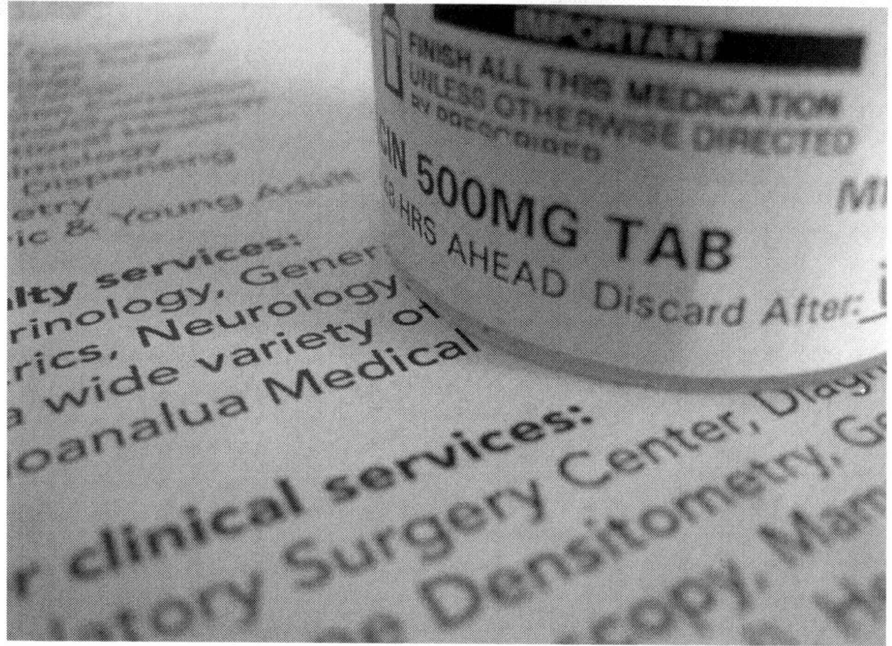

In this section, we'll review a number of individual antibiotics, delineating the indications, dosage, regimen, side effects, and other important information. We will also discuss some of the dilemmas that face the caregiver in austere settings, especially with dosing.

It's important to note that the below represents basic information on drugs that can currently be obtained without a prescription. In parenthesis you will find U.S. brand names and the name of available veterinary equivalents. We include some thoughts on their use in truly austere settings; these should not be construed as advice for normal times.

It's important to know that dosing may vary for different illnesses. Specific dosing for every possible known infection is beyond the scope of a book this size (or three times the size, for that matter). Read the section on amoxicillin below to see what we mean.

We do, however, give adult dosage regimens for all the infections we mention in this book. Consult the references mentioned previously for a complete and comprehensive listing of dosing, side effects, and other considerations for every antibiotic and every infection.

INDICATIONS, DOSING, RISKS, AND SPECIAL CONSIDERATIONS

The management of antibiotic therapy is a daunting challenge for the average person in an austere setting. Without modern medicine, a caregiver must develop a fund of knowledge regarding each drug: its strengths, weaknesses, mechanism of action, and risks. Each drug differs in these and other characteristics. Misunderstanding antibiotics leads, in many cases, to more problems than not using the antibiotic at all.

To begin our discussion of individual antibiotics, we must understand some basic terms:

- **Indications:** the reason why you would use a particular drug.
- **Contraindications:** the reasons why you wouldn't use a particular drug.
- **Dosage**: the amount of drug appropriate for an individual's age, weight, and other factors.
- **Regimen**: a prescribed course of medical treatment or diet (or way of life, for that matter). An example might be: Amoxicillin 500mg orally every 8 hours for 7 days.

- **Side Effects:** reactions, usually negative, that occur as a result of taking a drug in a percentage of patients.
- **Interactions:** the change in the effect of a drug when using other medications or substances. The effect may be to increase its potency, decrease it, or cause a side effect of some sort.
- **Pregnancy category:** whether the medication is safe to use in pregnancy or during breastfeeding.
- **Veterinary equivalent:** the brand name of the medication in the version offered to the pet industry.
- **Special considerations:** Some antibiotics are recommended to take on an empty stomach and some with meals. Given that oral drugs and food end up in the same stomach, it makes sense that they can interact. It often comes down to the effect of stomach acid, which is highest when there is food to digest.

There are drugs that are best absorbed into the bloodstream when the environment in the gut is particularly acidic. Thus, taking these with food is the best approach.

So, what about the ones taken on an empty stomach? An empty stomach is defined as at least an hour before or two hours after a meal. If a drug is suggested to be taken without food, it may be because the chemical compound easily degrades in an acidic environment; penicillin V is an example.

It is well-known that some drugs, like Ibuprofen, may cause stomach irritation or nausea if taken on an empty stomach. Other drugs ingested with certain foods that contain iron, calcium, or other nutrients may be made more or less potent by them.

The terms we've just defined are so important that they deserve more explanation, which continues below.

Contraindications

Earlier, we defined an "**indication**" for a drug as the medical condition that would be cured or otherwise benefit from its use. This is opposed to a contraindicated drug. In medicine, a "**contraindication**" is some condition or factor that makes an action, such as administering a medicine, inadvisable (or even dangerous).

There are **absolute contraindications**: Situations where there is no circumstance you would use the antibiotic in question. For example, penicillin is an absolute contraindication in people who have had severe allergic reactions when given it in the past.

Relative contraindications are situations where there are dangers involved in a course of treatment, but the benefits outweigh the risks in certain situations. Normally, you wouldn't want to perform X-rays on pregnant woman but if a serious condition is suspected, the benefit of diagnosing it and beginning treatment may save her life.

In the forthcoming discussion of individual antibiotics, most have **broad spectrum** indications. The antibiotic may be useful against various bacterial species, bacteria and protozoa, and/or a large number of infections. Each will also have its share of adverse reactions, allergic potential, and contraindications, so proceed with caution.

Pregnancy

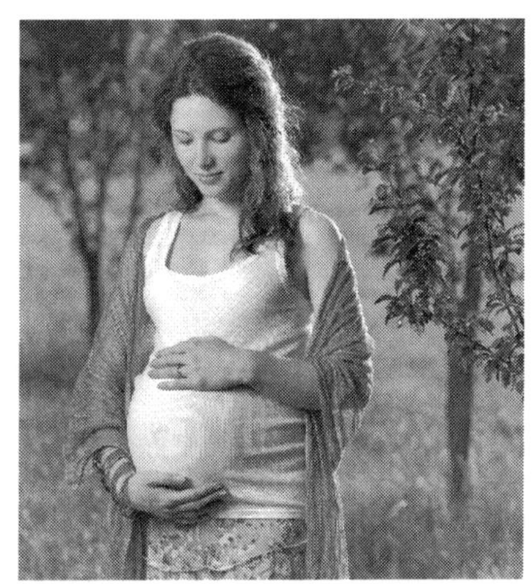

Besides allergies, there are other times when a particular antibiotic (or another drug) should not be used. Many medications, for example, are not recommended for use during pregnancy. Sometimes, this is because lab studies have shown birth defects in animal fetuses exposed to the drug. Other times, it is because no studies on pregnant women or animals have yet been performed. The latter is commonly the case, as there are many ethical considerations when it comes to testing drugs on people.

Despite the uncertainty of certain drugs' safety due to inadequate testing, the Food and Drug Administration (FDA) attempts to guide citizens on the safety of a drug during pregnancy or while breastfeeding.

In the past, FDA recommendations were based in the U.S. on a pregnancy category (usually a letter: A, B, C, D, X, N):

Category A
Adequate and well-controlled studies have failed to demonstrate a risk to the fetus in the first trimester of pregnancy (and there is no evidence of risk in later trimesters).

Category B
Animal reproduction studies have failed to demonstrate a risk to the fetus; there are no adequate and well-controlled studies in pregnant women.

Category C
Animal reproduction studies have shown an adverse effect on the fetus; there are no adequate and well-controlled studies in humans, but potential benefits may warrant use of the drug in pregnant women despite potential risks.

Category D
There is positive evidence of human fetal risk based on adverse reaction data from studies in humans or other data, but potential benefits may warrant use of the drug in pregnant women despite potential risks.

Category X
Studies in animals or humans have demonstrated fetal abnormalities and/or there is positive evidence of human fetal risk based on adverse reaction data from investigational or marketing experience; the risks involved in use of the drug on pregnant women clearly outweigh potential benefits.

Category N
Not yet classified.

Many countries have their own categories that differ slightly from the above. In 2015, the FDA replaced the old labeling system with new information considered more comprehensive. Instead of an assigned category, the new system gives a much more detailed narrative on each drug. It should be noted that drugs available before 2015 are allowed to slowly phase in the current more elaborate information. You may see many sites where the old categories are still used.

Whether the old, the new, or any of a number of international classifications are used, it remains true that a definitive answer is not often possible regarding the safety of many drugs during pregnancy and breastfeeding. Despite this, the austere medic should have a number of over-the-counter pregnancy tests as part of their medical storage.

Children

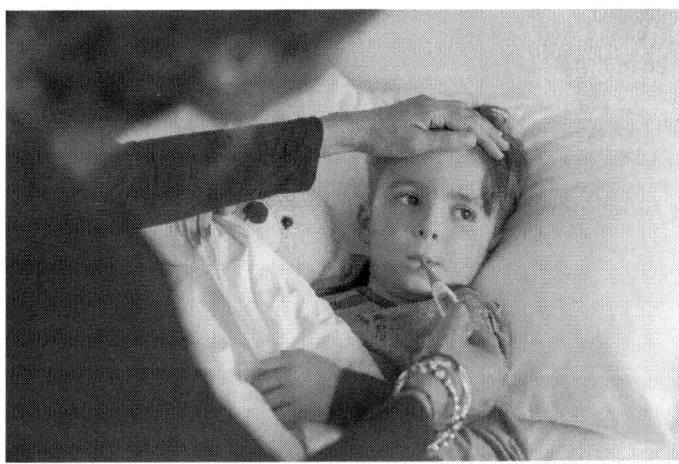

A child is not just a little adult

Adults aren't the only ones that can get infected by bacteria; children are also susceptible, especially to infections of the ear, throat, and upper respiratory tract. Although antibiotics may be needed, care should be taken; overuse is as major an issue with children as it is with adults. In one study, researchers estimated that, although only 27 percent of ear infections in children are caused by bacteria, 57 percent were given prescriptions for antibiotics.

It is a false assumption that children are just little adults. They are more vulnerable to the rapid spread of infectious diseases for several reasons:

- Their immune systems are immature.
- They are naturally curious and more apt to handle contaminated items.
- They are more likely to put fingers and objects in their mouths.
- They have not completed vaccination schedules.
- They breathe more often per minute than adults, possibly increasing the chance of inhaling air droplets containing pathogens.
- They have less body fluid reserves and become dehydrated more easily.
- They are dependent on others for their care.

There are also differences in body size, metabolism, the progress of disease, and, of course, age that often cause a different response to the drug. It may be absorbed, metabolized, or eliminated faster or slower, with variable end results.

As such, expect dosages for children to be different that those for adults. Indeed, you will find that some antibiotics are forbidden in children altogether. We'll illustrate the variations regarding pediatric dosages for different infections when we discuss the antibiotic amoxicillin and others later in the book.

Chronic Medical Illness

Some drugs are risky if used on individuals with chronic medical issues. Those with kidney or liver disease, for example, may have difficulty excreting or metabolizing certain antibiotics. This may cause drug effects to be greater than desired or have more severe adverse reactions.

The medic should consider themselves archivists of the medical histories of all for whom they are responsible. Knowledge of each patient's medical, surgical, allergy, and medication history is essential to be effective in keeping them healthy. For a more extensive discussion, see our book "The Survival Medicine Handbook: The Essential Guide for when Medical Help is Not on the Way."

Drug Interactions

An additional circumstance where a particular medication should not be used is the possible adverse interaction of multiple drugs or substances used at the same time. For example, taking the antibiotic metronidazole and drinking alcohol could make you vomit. Grapefruit juice taken with statin drugs may increase your chance of liver and muscle damage.

Some drug interactions may cause the effect of one of them to become stronger or weaker. A certain medicine, for example, may decrease the effect of another when taken together.

"The Drug Of Choice"

As mentioned earlier, specific antibiotics are used for different infections, and it is important to know which medication is best for each infection. Indeed, every infection has a "drug of choice" that is the "first line" antibiotic you should use whenever possible. Others that can be used are often referred to as "second line." Unfortunately, some of these antibiotics won't be featured here as they might be intravenous in nature, or just not easily available to be an option for the average caregiver in an austere setting.

Let's take an example: Otitis media is an ear infection often seen in children. Amoxicillin is one of the "drugs of choice" for this condition. That is, it is recommended as a first line when you make this particular diagnosis (as long as the patient is not allergic to it). The drug of choice for a particular ailment may change, over time, based on new scientific evidence.

What happens if your patient is allergic to Amoxicillin? Before administering this (or any) medication, you should always take a full history including any episodes of allergies or adverse reactions to medicines. The most common form of allergy would appear as a rash, but swelling, itchiness, and even respiratory difficulty could occur. If you see any of these symptoms, you should discontinue your treatment, administer epinephrine (Epi-Pen or other auto-injector), and look for other options.

As with any medical emergency, seek professional help if available.

In the above case of an ear infection, antibiotics such as Azithromycin or Sulfamethoxazole/Trimethoprim could be a "second-line" solution.

It should be noted that there is always some variance when you receive opinions about treatment from different caregivers. Physicians often have a personal preference as to which drug they will use to treat a certain infection. They may not match the antibiotics listed here.

This book discusses only medications available for use in austere settings. They are often not the drug of choice; in some cases, the preferred treatment is only given intravenously. Let's face it, choices are more limited to the austere medic than for a specialist at a big-city hospital. When a drug will work against a certain disease, we will list it even if it is not the drug of choice or first line treatment.

Later in this section, we will review each antibiotic available to the family medic in some detail.

ANTIBIOTICS AVAILABLE TO THE AUSTERE MEDIC

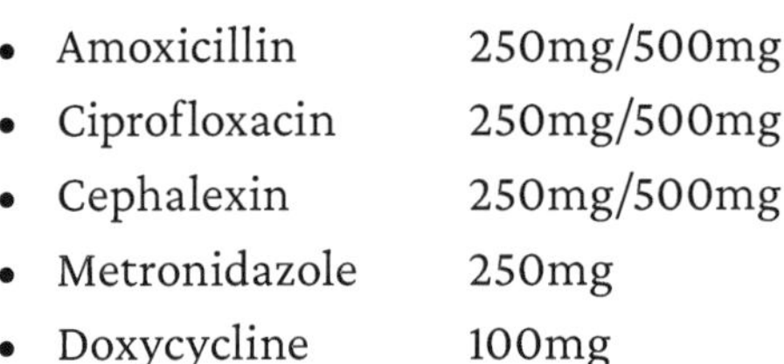

Antibiotics must be used properly to be effective. There are many to choose from, but what antibiotics accessible to the average person would be good additions to your medical storage? When do you use a particular drug? In this section, we'll discuss antibiotics you will want in your medical arsenal. They include (veterinary equivalent names in parentheses):

- Amoxicillin 250mg/500mg
- Ciprofloxacin 250mg/500mg
- Cephalexin 250mg/500mg
- Metronidazole 250mg
- Doxycycline 100mg
- Minocycline 50 mg/100mg
- Ampicillin 250mg/500mg
- Sulfamethoxazole 400mg/Trimethoprim 80mg
- Clindamycin 150mg
- Azithromycin 250mg
- Penicillin 250mg/500mg
- Fluconazole 100mg
- Ketoconazole 200mg

The above medications all come in capsules, tablets, or dosed powder packets, and are for oral use; you may see them referred to as "PO" drugs from the Latin "Per Oral." There is enough variety that even those with Penicillin allergies have several options (listed earlier). Intravenous medications are not discussed in any detail in this book due to the difficulty in obtaining them in any quantity without a prescription.

Some have asked how to turn oral medications into intravenous ones. While a solution of a drug can be made by mixing with water or saline solution, there are serious sterility concerns when you consider placing it directly into someone's veins. If the solution is not completely sterile, it is possible that you are giving your patient an infection worse than the one you're treating (and you're injecting it right into their bloodstream). The end result could be fatal.

We are often asked about veterinary antibiotics other than the ones mentioned above. There are many other meds that might be used on dogs and other animals, like Clavamox, that are essentially the same as a human antibiotic (Amoxicillin with clavulanate potassium, brand name Augmentin). The problem with small mammal antibiotics (or large mammal antibiotics, for that matter) is that the dosage of the drug is not one that easily translates into a human dosage.

You can imagine that horse or bovine meds are likely an overdose for a human. Small animal drugs present a different problem: For example, the dosage in canines is 6.25 mg/lb. twice a day. For adult humans, the dose is often 875 mg twice a day. The dog version (Clavamox) comes in 62mg, 125mg, 250mg, and 375mg. Although it's possible to extrapolate, it's much simpler to work with drugs produced exactly in the dosages used by humans.

Amoxicillin

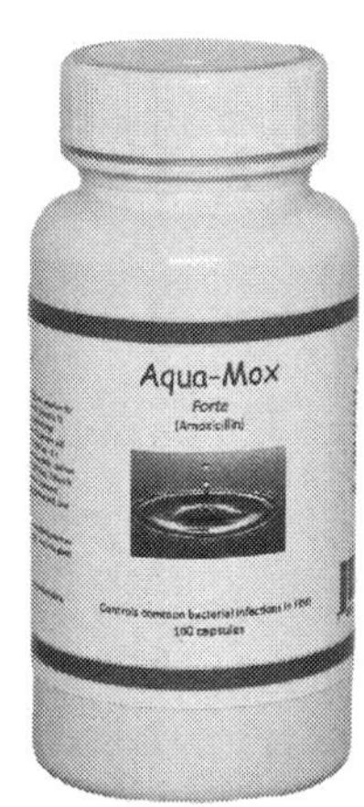

Amoxicillin is a member of the beta-lactam (penicillin) family of drugs: comes in 250mg and 500mg doses, usually taken 3 times a day. The "human version," marketed by the brand name Amoxil, also comes in 875mg doses taken twice a day. Amoxicillin is the most common antibiotic prescribed to children, usually in the form of liquid suspensions.

Amoxicillin acts similarly to penicillin in that it kills susceptible bacteria during the stage of active multiplication. It accomplishes this goal by inhibiting cell wall synthesis at a critical step. The faulty finished product is fragile and bursts easily, killing the bacterium. Although it is "bactericidal," the drug doesn't interfere with any function or process that goes on in humans. As such, it is generally considered safe and used for many infections.

Amoxicillin is tolerated well by patients, and is more versatile and better absorbed than the older penicillins. It is acceptable for use during pregnancy. Penicillin, ampicillin, and cephalexin, featured later, are related drugs.

Amoxicillin may be used for non-resistant organisms causing the following diseases (adult doses in parenthesis):

- **Cutaneous anthrax prevention or treatment**
  - » (1 g orally every 8 hours for 60 days)
- **Chlamydia**
  - » (500 mg orally 3 times a day for 7 days)
- **Gonorrhea**
  - » (3 grams in a single dose)
- **Bladder or kidney infections**
  - » (500 mg orally every 8-12 hours for 7 days)

- **Lyme disease**
  - » (500 mg orally every 8 hours for 14-28 days)
- **Otitis media**
  - » (Adult dose: 500 mg orally 3 times a day x 5-7 days)
  - » (Pediatric dose: 80-90 mg/kg/day orally in 2 divided doses for 7-10 days; never exceed adult dosages)
- **Bronchitis caused by bacteria**
  - » (500 mg orally 3 times a day for minimum of 5 days or until no fever for 2-3 days)
- **Pneumonia caused by bacteria**
  - » (500-1000 mg orally 3 times a day for minimum of 5 days or until no fever for 2-3 days)
- **Sinusitis**
  - » (250-500 mg orally 3 times a day for 5-7 days)
- **Skin or soft tissue infections like cellulitis**
  - » (250-500 mg orally 3 times a day for 7-10 days)
- **Tonsillitis/Pharyngitis** (Group A Strep throat)
  - » (1000 mg orally once a day or 500 mg orally twice a day for 10 days)
- **Mastitis (breast infection)**
  - » (500 mg orally 3 times a day for 10-14 days)

For most infections in adults, 500 mg of amoxicillin three times a day for 7-14 days is the usual treatment **regimen**. As you can see, with every antibiotic there is variation in dosage and length of therapy based on the disease.

Besides the dosages that come in veterinary equivalents, human antibiotics often have additional dosing options. For example, amoxicillin has an 875 mg dosage available in the human version. This may be more convenient, as the higher dose allows the medicine to be taken twice a day rather than three times. In severe infections, the higher dose may be suggested as the best alternative. Note that pediatric doses should never exceed adult doses regardless of the weight of the child.

Pediatric dosages are based upon weight in most cases and are even more varied. A common older child's dosage would be 250 mg two or three times a day. If you have tablets, you might have to break one in half; some open the capsule to separate out a portion that would be appropriate. This is an option only in austere settings or when directed by a qualified medical professional.

For amoxicillin, you would give a pediatric dose of 20-50 mg per kilogram (1 kilogram = 2.2 pounds) of body weight. For infants less than four months old, the dosage is 20-30 mg per kilogram.

To illustrate the variation that exists in recommended dosing, here's official pediatric dosing recommendations for amoxicillin from drugs.com for just one medical issue: skin and soft tissue infections:

"Mild, Moderate, or Severe Infection:

- 3 months or younger: Up to 30 mg/kg/day orally in divided doses every 12 hours
  - » Treatment should be continued for a minimum of 48 to 72 hours beyond the time the patient becomes asymptomatic or evidence of bacterial eradication occurs.
  - » At least 10 days of treatment for any infection caused by *Streptococcus pyogenes* is recommended to prevent the occurrence of acute rheumatic fever.

Mild to Moderate Infection:

- 4 months or older:
  - » Less than 40 kg: 20 mg/kg/day orally in divided doses every 8 hours or 25 mg/kg/day in divided doses every 12 hours
  - » At least 40 kg: 250 mg orally every 8 hours or 500 mg every 12 hours

Severe Infection:

- 4 months or older:
  - » Less than 40 kg: 40 mg/kg/day orally in divided doses every 8 hours or 45 mg/kg/day in divided doses every 12 hours
  - » At least 40 kg: 500 mg orally every 8 hours or 875 mg every 12 hours"

Here you see the recommendations are different for infants 3 months or younger, those 4 months or older weighing less than 40 kilograms, those 4 months or older weighing more than 40 kilograms, and those with mild, moderate, and severe infection.

Add to that the dozens of infections that amoxicillin treats, you can see the difficulty in presenting all of this information in a book this size. As such, we give the most common doses that treat many infections.

If your child is too young to swallow a pill whole, you can make a mixture with water (called a "**suspension**"). To make a liquid suspension, crush a tablet or empty a capsule of the appropriate dosage into a small glass of water or juice. Shake well and drink it with or without food. Then, fill again to get the particles that may adhere to the walls of the glass and drink. Many add flavoring of some sort to make it taste better.

Do not chew or make a suspension out of time-released capsules of any medication; you will wind up losing some of the gradual release effect and perhaps get too much into your system at once. These medications are usually plainly marked "Time-Released" or "Extended-Release."

Amoxicillin is acceptable to take with or without meals. Common side effects include stomach upset, diarrhea, headache, and dizziness. Avoid using in those who are allergic to penicillin.

Amoxicillin is considered generally safe for use during pregnancy or breastfeeding. Infants may develop oral yeast infections called "thrush" or diarrhea in response to the mother's antibiotic use during breastfeeding.

Amoxicillin has issues related to growing bacterial resistance. A combination of amoxicillin and clavulanic acid (known as Augmentin) is more effective against resistant bacteria and available orally. The small animal antibiotic Clavamox is the same medication and counters some of these concerns, but does not come in human dosages. Thus, it wouldn't be as simple to dose correctly.

Ampicillin

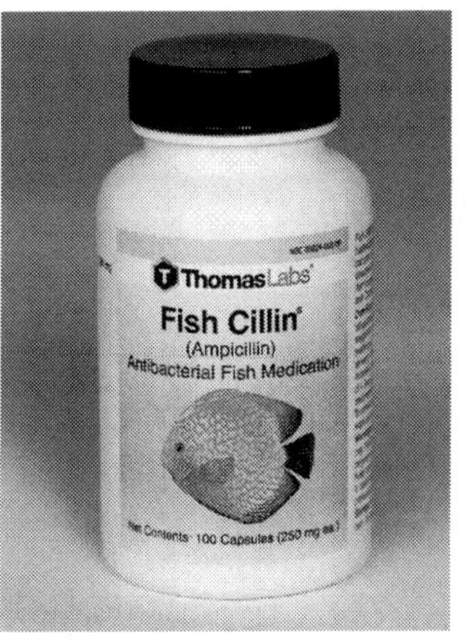

Ampicillin is a member of the penicillin (beta-lactam) family. It is bactericidal due to its ability to interfere with bacteria cell walls. Ampicillin can be used to treat a number of bacterial infections:

- **Respiratory tract Infections caused by bacteria**
  - » (250-500 mg orally every 6 hours for 5-10 days)
- **Throat infections caused by bacteria**
  - » (250-500 mg orally every 6 hours for 5-10 days)
- **Ear infections**
  - » (500 mg orally every 6 hours for 7-10 days)
- **Sinusitis**
  - » (250-500 mg orally every 6 hours for 7-10 days)
- **Skin and soft tissue infections like cellulitis**
  - » (250-500 mg orally every 6 hours)
- **Meningitis caused by bacteria**
  - » (150-200 mg/kg/day IV in equally divided doses every 3- 4 hours; an example of a disease not effectively treated with oral medication)

- **Bladder infections (cystitis)**
  - » (500 mg orally every 6 hours for 7 days)
- **Kidney infections** (pyelonephritis)
  - » (500 mg orally every 6 hours for 14-28 days)
- **Typhoid fever** (*Salmonella typhi* infection)
  - » (500 mg orally every 6 hours for 10-14 days)
- **Dysentery** (*Shigella* infection)
  - » (500 mg orally every 6 hours for 5 days)
- **Ear infections**
  - » (500 mg orally every 6 hours for 5-7 days)
- **Gastro-intestinal tract infections due to bacteria**
  - » (500 mg orally every 6 hours for 10-14 days)

Ampicillin is usually given to adults in doses of 250-500 mg 4 times a day for 7-10 days. A common pediatric dosage formula for infants over one month of age is 6.25-12.5 mg/kg every 6 hours (not to exceed adult dosages).

Take ampicillin on an empty stomach with a full glass of water at least one hour before or two hours after a meal.

Ampicillin is acceptable for use during pregnancy. Like most antibiotics, it has stronger effect in intravenous form, and is used IV in some cases of septicemia (blood infection) and endocarditis (heart infection).

Ampicillin may cause diarrhea, stomach upset, headache, nausea, and itching. Ampicillin should not be taken by those with allergies to penicillin or cephalosporin family drugs.

It should be noted that, due to bacterial resistance, Ampicillin has been supplanted in many instances by ampicillin/sulbactam (Unasyn, Sultamicillin). Sulbactam is added to counteract a chemical produced by resistant bacteria called beta-lactamase. Unfortunately, ampicillin/sulbactam is not available in a veterinary equivalent.

Penicillin

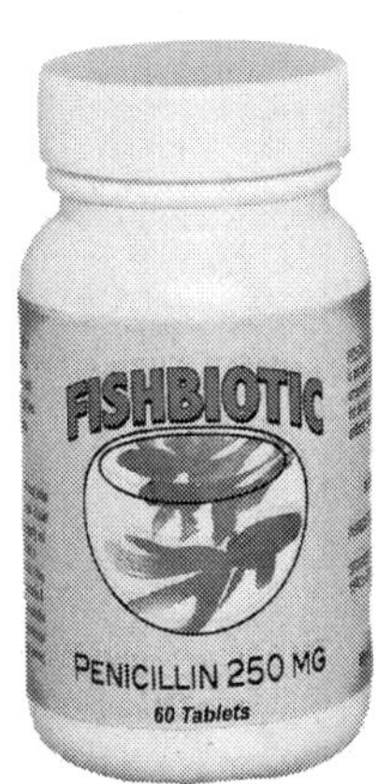

One of the most important and earliest antibiotics, penicillin is a bactericidal antibiotic effective mostly against gram-positive organisms. It has been supplanted by newer generations of the penicillin (also called "Beta-Lactam") family due to serious problems with bacterial resistance.

Penicillin may still be an option to treat:

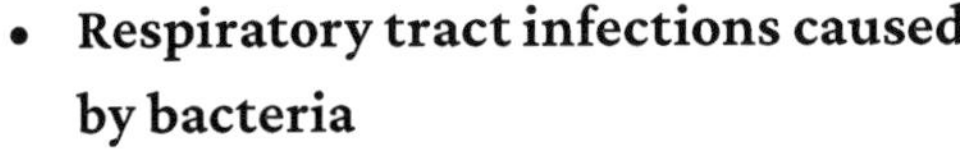

- **Respiratory tract infections caused by bacteria**
  - » (250-500 mg orally every 6 hours until no fever for at least 2 days)
- **Skin or soft tissue infection like cellulitis**
  - » (250-500 mg orally every 6- 8 hours until no signs noted)
- **Tonsillitis or pharyngitis**
  - » (500 mg orally 2 to 3 times a day for 10 days)
- **Scarlet fever**
  - » (250 mg orally every 6-8 hours for 10 days)
- **Cutaneous (skin-related) anthrax**
  - » (500 mg orally every 6 hours for 10 days; 60 if bioterror-related)
- **Joint infections caused by bacteria**
  - » (500 mg orally 2-4 times a day for 2-6 weeks)
- **Ear infections like otitis media**
  - » (250-500 mg orally every 6 hours for 10 days or until patient afebrile for at least 2 days)
- **Dental infections**
  - » (250-500 mg orally every 6 hours for 3 days; if no improvement, re-examine)

Adult dosing is usually in the 250-500 mg range every 6-8 hours for 10 days. Pediatric doses for children over 12 years of age are usually in the 125-500 mg range every 6-8 hours. For infants and other young children 1 month or older: 25-75 mg/kg/day in oral suspension (see amoxicillin section) in 3 or 4 divided doses. Pediatric dosages should not exceed adult dosages.

Common adverse reactions include diarrhea, nausea, rash, hives, and secondary infections with fungi.

Penicillin use is considered acceptable during pregnancy, and likely safe for use in breastfeeding mothers. Users should be alert to allergic reaction symptoms like difficulty breathing, rashes, and swelling. Like many drugs in this family, the possibility of resistance should be a concern.

Cephalexin

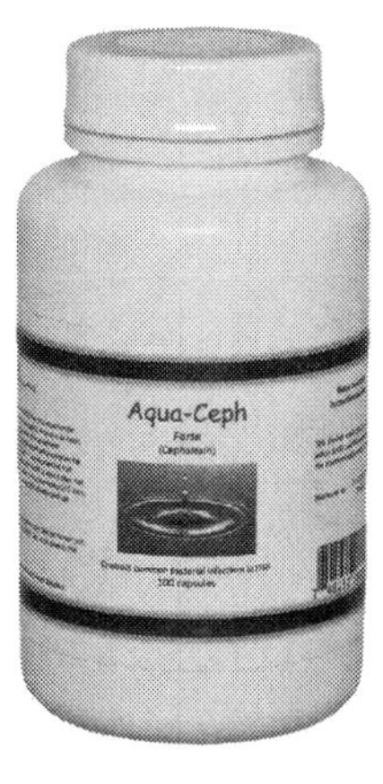

Cephalexin is an antibiotic in the Cephalosporin family, one of various that are classified as "Beta-Lactams." The drug is marketed in the U.S. under the name "Keflex."

Cephalosporins kill gram-positive and some gram-negative bacteria in a fashion similar to penicillins: By disrupting the growth of the bacterial cell wall. This causes the defective wall to rupture, killing the bacteria. Cephalexin is one of the earlier cephalosporins and is considered "first-generation." A number of drugs in the same family have been introduced since then, but cephalexin (Keflex) is one of the few available in veterinary form.

Cephalosporins are different from, but cross-reactive with, the Penicillin family. It is thought that 10% or more of penicillin-allergic patients will also exhibit an allergy to cephalosporins.

Cephalexin is useful in the treatment of infections caused by bacteria in the following areas:

- **Pyelonephritis** (kidney infections), **cystitis** (bladder infections) or **prostate infections**
  - » (250 mg orally every 6 hours or 500 mg every 12 hours for 7 days)
- **Ear infections like otitis media**
  - » (250 orally every 6 hours or 500 mg every 12 hours for 7-14 days)
- **Pharyngitis** (throat infections)
  - » (250 orally every 6 hours or 500 mg every 12 hours for 7-14 days)
- **Soft tissue infection** (cellulitis)
  - » (500 mg orally every 6 hours for 7-14 days)
- **Skin infections** (impetigo)
  - » (250 mg orally every 6 hours for 7-14 days)
- **Osteomyelitis** (infections of bone and marrow)
  - » (500 mg orally every 6-12 hours for 4-6 weeks)
- **Upper respiratory tract infections caused by bacteria**
  - » (250 mg orally every 6 hours or 500 mg every 12 hours for 7-14 days)
- **Mastitis**
  - » (500 mg every 6 hours for 10-14 days)

Cephalexin is also used as a preventative before some dental and surgical procedures, especially in people who are diabetics, have weak immune systems, or are at risk for heart or other blood-borne infections. Often, the treatment consists of one or two doses a few hours before the procedure.

As treatment for most infections, you would normally give adults or children over 15 years of age 250 mg cephalexin every 6 hours or 500 mg every 12 hours for 7-14 days. Severe cases may require an additional week of therapy. Infections of the bone (osteomyelitis) are particularly dangerous and require 4-6 weeks of therapy. More modern cephalosporins that can be given intravenously are commonly used in the more severe infections.

Cephalexin is used in infants and children to treat the same infections seen in adults. Pediatric dosages are calculated using 12.5 to 25 mg per kilogram of body weight orally every 6-12 hours for 7-14 days (never exceed adult dosages).

Although cephalexin may be taken with or without meals, those with sensitive stomachs should ingest it with a full glass of water during a meal.

Cephalexin is considered to be a pregnancy category B drug using the old classification system. It has not been shown to cause fetal defects in animal studies. It may be used during pregnancy and breastfeeding at standard doses. As a matter of fact, it is used as a treatment for a cellulitis of the breast called "**mastitis**" seen in breastfeeding mothers.

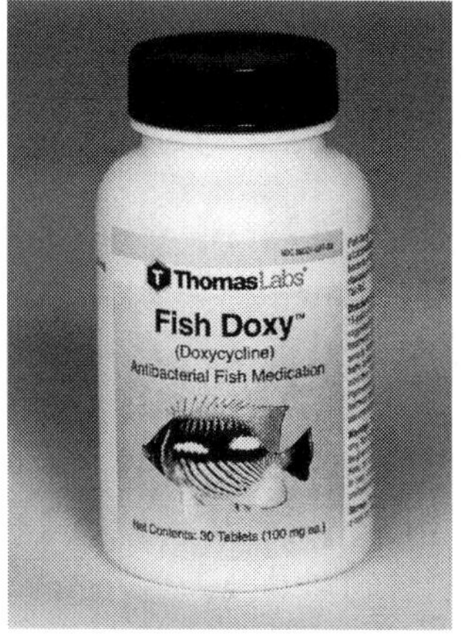

Doxycycline

Doxycycline is a member of the broad-spectrum tetracycline family. In recent years, it has seen much more use than its older relative tetracycline. Like other members of its class, doxycycline prevents microbe reproduction by inhibiting the manufacture of bacterial proteins.

Doxycycline is an example where the veterinary version often comes in dosed powder packets instead of capsules or tablets. It is still the exact dose to use in adult humans.

Doxycycline is an extraordinarily versatile drug. Indications for its usage include the following:

- **Diarrheal disease caused by E. coli, Shigella, Listeria, Campylobacter, Entamoeba, and other "food poisoning" or dysentery-like infections**
  - » (100 mg orally every 12 hours the first day, followed by 50-100 mg once or twice daily for 10 days)
- **Chlamydia** (sexually transmitted disease)

   » (100 mg every 12 hours for 7 days; an extended-release doxycycline may be acceptable as single dose therapy)
- **Gonorrhea**
   » (100 mg orally every 12 hours for 7 days; alternatively, 300 mg orally followed in 1 hour by a second 300 mg)
- **Syphilis** (latent, primary, or secondary)
   » (Primary or secondary syphilis: 100 mg orally twice a day for 14 days; Latent: 100 mg orally twice a day for 28 days)
- **Lyme disease** (tick-borne)
   » (100 mg orally every 12 hours the first day, followed by 50-100 mg once or twice daily for 10 days)
- **Rocky Mountain spotted fever** (tick-borne)
   » (100 mg orally every 12 hours the first day, followed by 50-100 mg once or twice daily for 10 days)
- **Inhalational anthrax**
   » (100 mg every 12 hours for 60 days)
- **Cholera**
   » (100 mg orally every 12 hours the first day, followed by 50-100 mg once or twice daily for 10 days)
- **Typhus**
   » (100 mg orally every 12 hours the first day, followed by 50-100 mg once or twice daily for 10 days)
- **Plague**
   » (100 mg orally every 12 hours the first day, followed by 50-100 mg once or twice daily for 10 days)
- **Dental infections**
   » (100mg every 12 hours on the first day, followed by 100mg once daily for 21 days)
- **Hidradenitis suppurativa, boils, abscesses, acne and other skin conditions characterized by infection**

  - » (100 mg orally every 12 hours the first day, followed by 50-100 mg once or twice daily for 10 days)
- **Urinary tract infections**
  - » (100 mg orally every 12 hours the first day, followed by 50-100 mg once or twice daily for 10 days)
- **Respiratory infections caused by bacteria** (including bronchitis and pneumonia)
  - » (100 mg orally every 12 hours the first day, followed by 50-100 mg once or twice daily for 10 days)
- **Methicillin-resistant Staph (MRSA) infections**
  - » (100 mg orally every 12 hours for 10 days or longer)
- **Necrotizing fasciitis**
  - » (100 mg orally every 12 hours for 10 days or longer)
- **Malaria** (prevention)
  - » (100 mg orally once a day during exposure; with quinine, may serve as a treatment if taken every 12 hours for 7 days)
- **Periodontal disease and gingivitis** (gum and oral soft tissues)

In the case of Rocky Mountain spotted fever, doxycycline is indicated for use even in children. Otherwise, doxycycline is not meant for those under the age of eight years. It has not been approved for use during pregnancy but is considered "probably safe" for short-term use in breastfeeding mothers.

The recommended doxycycline dosage for most types of bacterial infections in adults is 100 mg to 200 mg per day for 7-14 days. For chronic (long-term) or more serious infections, treatment can be carried out for a longer time. For example, anthrax victims should receive treatment for 60 days. In the rare cases that it is appropriate, children will receive 1-2 mg per pound of body weight per day, usually divided into two doses.

Some dental infections, if severe, may merit treatment with doxycycline 100 mg orally every 12 hours the first day, followed by 100 mg once daily for 21 days thereafter.

If the medication comes as a capsule, swallow it whole with water. Doxycycline that comes in dose packets of powder may be sprinkled onto cold, soft food like applesauce. Avoid stomach upset by not laying down soon after taking.

Doxycycline can be used as a preventative against malaria by taking 100 mg once a day in high-risk areas. Begin one to two days before arriving and continue for four weeks after returning.

Side-effects include nausea and vomiting, diarrhea, rash, and loss of appetite. Like all tetracyclines, doxycycline is acceptable for use in penicillin-allergic patients. It is contraindicated, however, in pregnancy and breastfeeding. Resistance to doxycycline is becoming an issue, but not as much as older drugs.

Minocycline

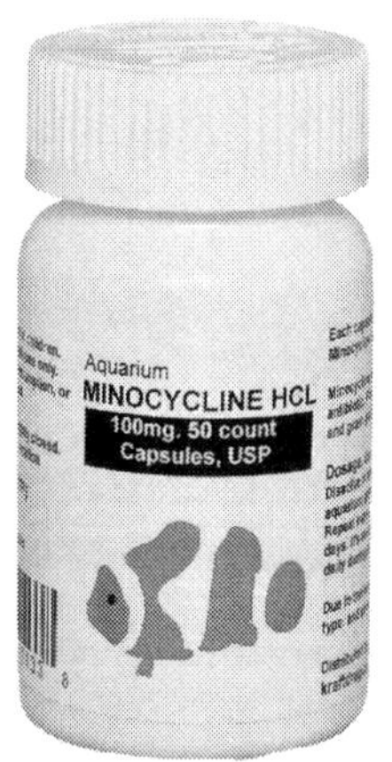

Minocycline is a bacteriostatic antibiotic in the Tetracycline family of drugs. It inhibits the ability of bacteria to synthesize important proteins needed for growth and reproduction. Minocycline differs from older class members in that it remains in higher concentrations in the body for longer periods of time.

Minocycline has been used to treat the following infections:

- **Diarrheal disease caused by E. coli, Enterobacter, Campylobacter, Acinetobacter, Entamoeba, Shigella, and other "food poisoning" or dysentery-like infections**
  - » (100 mg orally every 12 hours the first day, followed by 50-100 mg once or twice daily for 10 days)
- **Chlamydia** (sexually transmitted disease)
  - » (100 mg orally every 12 hours for at least 7 days)

- **Gonorrhea**
    - » (100 mg orally every 12 hours for 5 days if urethra is inflamed; otherwise, 200 mg orally once followed by 100 mg every 12 hours for at least 4 days)
- **Pelvic inflammatory disease caused by STDs**
    - » (Doxycycline 100 mg orally twice daily for 14 days)
- **Syphilis** (latent, primary, or secondary)
    - » (100 mg orally every 12 hours the first day, followed by 50-100 mg for 10-15 days)
- **Lyme disease** (tick-borne)
    - » (100 mg orally every 12 hours the first day, followed by 50-100 mg once or twice daily for 10 days)
- **Rocky Mountain spotted fever** (tick-borne)
    - » (100 mg orally every 12 hours the first day, followed by 50-100 mg once or twice daily for 10 days)
- **Inhalational anthrax**
    - » (100 mg every 12 hours for 60 days)
- **Cholera**
    - » (100 mg orally every 12 hours the first day, followed by 50-100 mg once or twice daily for 10 days)
- **Typhus**
    - » (100 mg orally every 12 hours the first day, followed by 50-100 mg once or twice daily for 10 days)

- **Plague**
  - » (100 mg orally every 12 hours the first day, followed by 50-100 mg once or twice daily for 10 days)
- **Hidradenitis suppurativa, boils, abscesses, acne and other skin conditions characterized by infection**
  - » (100 mg orally every 12 hours the first day, followed by 50-100 mg once or twice daily for 10 days)
- **Urinary tract infections**
  - » (100 mg orally every 12 hours the first day, followed by 50-100 mg once or twice daily for 10 days)
- **Respiratory infections caused by bacteria** (including bronchitis and pneumonia)
  - » (100 mg orally every 12 hours the first day, followed by 50-100 mg once or twice daily for 10 days)
- **Abscesses caused by methicillin-resistant Staph (MRSA) infections**
  - » (100 mg orally every 12 hours the first day, followed by 50-100 mg once or twice daily for 10 days)
- **Necrotizing fasciitis**
  - » (100 mg orally every 12 hours for 10 days or longer)
- **Respiratory infections** caused by *Mycoplasma pneumoniae, Hemophilus influenza,* and *Klebsiella* species
  - » (100 mg orally every 12 hours the first day, followed by 50-100 mg once or twice daily for 10 days)
- **Acne**
  - » (50 mg once daily for no longer than 12 weeks)

For most infections, a "**loading dose**" of 200 mg orally is initially given, followed by 100 mg every 12 hours for at least 7 days. An alternative regimen starts with 100 to 200 mg as a first dose, followed by 50 mg 4 times a day. For acne, dosage is determined by weight; use approximately 1 mg per kilogram once daily for 12 weeks.

Minocycline is not used in children under eight years of age. After eight years old, use 4 mg/kg orally once followed by 2 mg/kg every 12 hours for at least 7 days. Do not exceed adult dosages.

Take this medicine with a full glass of water; It can be taken at mealtime if desired. Swallow the drug whole if it's "time-released," as it is manufactured to be released slowly in the GI tract; chewing it would possibly cause too much of an effect all at once. Medications that are extended-release usually say so on the label.

Avoid antacids, laxatives, multivitamins, and supplements that contain calcium, magnesium, or iron as they can decrease the absorption of Minocycline.

Minocycline is not considered safe for use during pregnancy. It and other tetracyclines can cause fetal malformations and discoloration of tooth enamel. Short term use only is acceptable in breastfeeding mothers. Like many antibiotics, doses require a downward adjustment in those with kidney or liver disease.

Minocycline and its relatives are considered acceptable for use in those allergic to Penicillin family drugs.

Sulfa Drugs

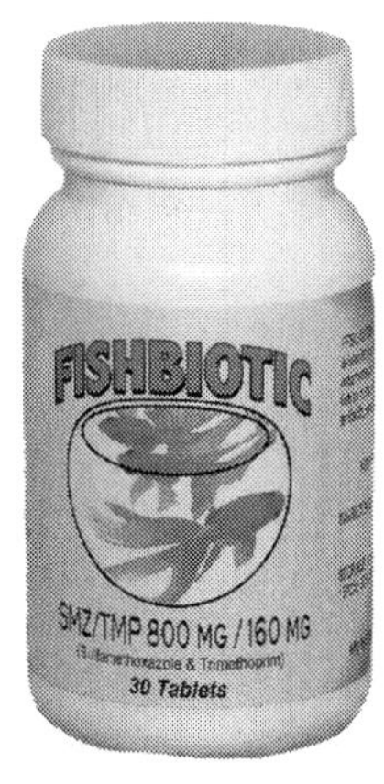

Sulfa drugs, also called sulfonamides, are bacteriostatic antibiotics that trace their lineage back to the 19th Century. Today, a popular descendant is a combination of two medications, sulfamethoxazole 400 mg and trimethoprim 80 mg. This drug, commonly written as SMX-TMP, eliminates a broad spectrum of gram-positive and gram-negative bacterial infections and is well-known commercially in the United States as Bactrim or

Septra. A double strength version known as "Bactrim DS" or "Septra DS" is also available.

Sulfamethoxazole acts as an inhibitor of an important bacterial enzyme; trimethoprim interferes with the production of folic acid in bacteria, which is necessary to produce DNA. Given in combination, laboratory studies show the two antibiotics together are stronger in their effect than if given separately.

Sulfamethoxazole 400mg/trimethoprim 80mg is effective in the treatment of the following:

- **Kidney** (pyelonephritis) and **bladder** (cystitis) **infections**
  - » (Sulfamethoxazole-trimethoprim 800 mg-160 mg orally every 12 hours for 10 to 14 days)
- **Ear infections** (otitis media)
  - » (Sulfamethoxazole-trimethoprim 800 mg-160 mg orally every 12 hours for 10 to 14 days)
- **Bronchitis caused by Hemophilus influenza and Streptococcus pneumoniae**
  - » (Sulfamethoxazole-trimethoprim 800 mg-160 mg orally every 12 hours for 14 days)
- **Traveler's diarrhea, dysentery and other intestinal infections caused by** E. Coli **and** Shigella **bacteria**
  - » (Sulfamethoxazole-trimethoprim 800 mg-160 mg orally every 12 hours for 5 days)
- **Skin and wound infections**
  - » (Some topical creams contain sulfadiazine, another sulfa drug mixed with silver in the product known as "Silvadene." It is used effectively for bedsores and a number of other wounds)

- **Acne**
  - » (Sulfamethoxazole-trimethoprim 800 mg-160 mg orally every 12 hours for 14 days in severe cases)
- **Certain MRSA infections**
  - » (Not FDA approved, but consider Sulfamethoxazole-trimethoprim 800 mg-160 mg orally every 12 hours for 10 to 14 days)
- **Sinusitis**
  - » (Sulfamethoxazole-trimethoprim 800 mg-160 mg orally every 12 hours for 2-4 weeks)
- **Cystitis prevention**
  - » (Sulfamethoxazole-trimethoprim 400 mg-80 mg orally once a day or 3 times a week at bedtime)

Sulfonamides are also components of some **topical** (skin) medications used to treat vaginal infections and as infection prevention for bedsores and burns. It should be noted that some sulfonamides have activity against certain fungal organisms. A recent study suggests that SMX-TMP may have potential in the treatment of malaria.

The usual dosage of SMX-TMP is two regular strength (SMX 400mg-TMP 80mg) tablets or one double strength (SMX 800mg/TMP 160mg) tablet twice a day in adults for 10-14 days (5 days in traveler's diarrhea and similar illnesses). Some physicians feel that simple bladder infections can be treated with only 3 days of therapy.

The recommended dose for pediatric patients with urinary tract infections or acute otitis media is 8 mg/kg trimethoprim and 40 mg/kg sulfamethoxazole per 24 hours, given in two divided doses every 12 hours for 10 days. This medication should not be used in infants 2 months old or younger.

In rat studies, the use of this drug was shown to cause birth defects; therefore, it is not used during pregnancy nor breastfeeding.

SMX-TMP and other sulfa drugs are well known to cause allergic reactions in some individuals but are acceptable for use in those allergic to penicillin. Allergies to sulfonamides are almost as common as penicillin allergies.

Common side effects include skin rash, hives, diarrhea, nausea and vomiting and loss of appetite. Use of sulfa drugs (and many other antibiotics) are associated with the development of yeast infections. Use is risky, as it is with many antibiotics, in those who suffer from kidney or liver dysfunction.

Clindamycin

Clindamycin is part of the family of drugs called Lincosamide antibiotics. It is generally bacteriostatic and works by slowing or stopping the growth of bacteria. This antibiotic is a first line drug against bacteria that are anaerobic, which means that they thrive in the absence of oxygen. These are often seen in deep puncture-type wounds.

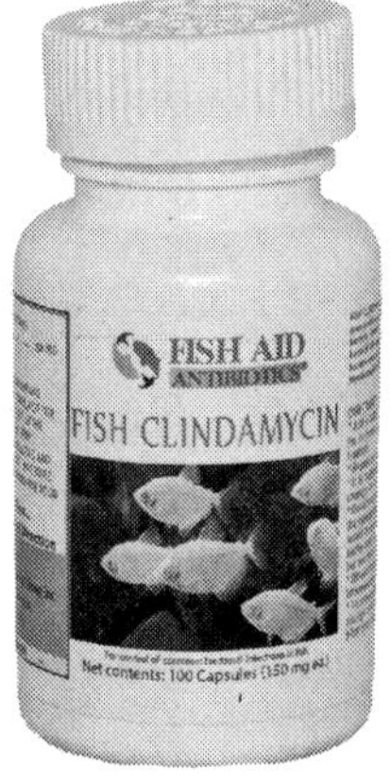

Clindamycin can be used to treat a number of infections:

- **Dental infections**
  - » (150 mg orally every 6 hours for 7 days)
- **Soft tissue infections** (cellulitis)
  - » (150-300 mg orally every 6 hours for 10 days)
- **Peritonitis** (inflammation of the abdominal lining)
  - » (150-300 mg orally every 6 hours for 10 days)
- **Pneumonia caused by** Strep, Staph, **or** Pneumococci
  - » (150-300 mg orally every 6 hours for 10 days; in the most severe cases, 300-450 mg orally every 6 hours)
- **Uterine infections** (such as after miscarriage or childbirth)
  - » (150-300 mg orally every 6 hours for 10 days)
- **Blood infections (septicemia)**,

    - » (IV meds are more effective. If unavailable, 300 to 450 mg orally every 6 hours may be an option)
- **Bite wounds** (animal or human)
    - » (300 mg orally every 6 hours for 10 days)
- **Pelvic inflammatory disease** (often caused by STDs)
    - » (150-300 mg orally every 6 hours for 10-14 days, often in combination with doxycycline 100 mg every 12 hours for 14 days)
- **Some MRSA** (Methicillin-resistant Staph. Aureus infections)
    - » (150-300 mg orally every 6 hours for 10 days)
- **Anthrax**
    - » (150-300 mg orally every 6 hours for 10 days or longer)
- **Malaria**
    - » (Only effective in conjunction with quinine, the combination can be used in children and is the treatment of choice for pregnant women in areas when resistance is common; 150 to 300 mg orally every 6 hours for 10 days)
- **Bacterial vaginosis**
    - » (300 mg orally every 12 hours for 7 days, but commonly used as a vaginal gel)

The length of therapy may vary based on the level of improvement and/or the appearance of serious adverse reactions to the GI tract or the liver.

Standard therapy with clindamycin consists of 150 mg or 300 mg doses every 6 hours. Pediatric dosage can be determined by body weight: If infants 10 kg or less, the recommended dose is 37.5 mg orally 3 times a day. For children with body weight 11 kg or greater, the formula is 8-12 mg/kg orally in 3 or 4 divided doses not to exceed adult dosages.

To avoid the possibility of irritation to the **esophagus**, administer clindamycin capsules with a full glass of water. Swallow capsules whole.

Clindamycin has shown no ill effects on the fetus in animal studies (old category B). With most drugs, testing cannot be done ethically on pregnant humans, so very few drugs are willing to say that they are completely safe during pregnancy. Breastfeeding may not be advisable, however, as the World Health Organization (WHO) reports that it can affect the good bacteria in the infant's gut.

Clindamycin is a viable option for use in patients with Penicillin allergies. This is not to say that you might not have a distinct allergy to clindamycin or any other antibiotic.

Common side effects include rash, abdominal cramps, nausea, and diarrhea. In addition, there is a serious diarrheal disease associated with Clindamycin use (and, although less so, many other antibiotics) caused by the overgrowth of a pathogen called *Clostridium difficile*. Symptoms may range in severity from mild diarrhea to fatal intestinal inflammation.

Because of this and risks to the liver and other organs, only use clindamycin for serious infections when absolutely necessary; discontinue any antibiotic that causes diarrhea, especially with blood or mucus, if at all possible.

Azithromycin

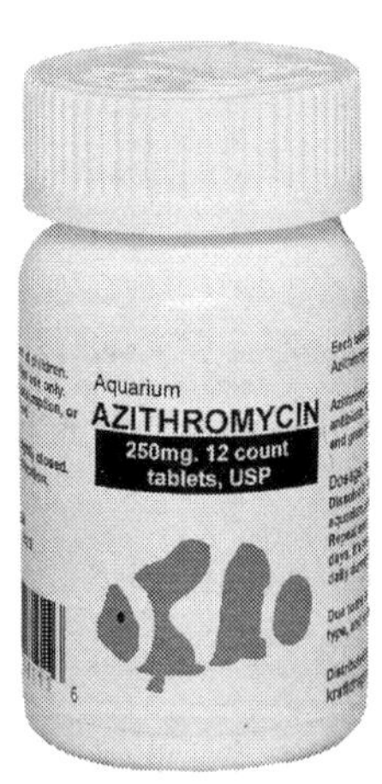

Azithromycin is a member of the generally bacteriostatic macrolide (erythromycin) family of antibiotics, although at higher doses, some macrolides work as a bactericide. Azithromycin interferes with bacteria's ability to make proteins necessary for growth and multiplication.

Azithromycin can be used to treat various types of:

- **Bronchitis caused by bacteria**
  - » (500 mg orally once daily for 3 days or 500 mg orally as a single dose on day 1, followed by 250 mg orally daily on days 2-5)
- **Pneumonia caused by Legionella, Hemophilus, Strep, mycoplasma, and others**
  - » (500 mg orally as a single dose on day 1, followed by 250 mg orally once a day on days 2 to 5)
- **Food poisoning caused by** Campylobacter
  - » (500 mg orally once a day for 5 days)
- **Dysentery caused by** Shigella
  - » (500 mg orally once a day for 5 days)
- **Skin infections**
  - » (500 mg orally as a single dose on day 1, followed by 250 mg orally once a day on days 2-5)
- **Throat infections caused by Group A Strep**
  - » (500 mg orally as a single dose on day 1, followed by 250 mg orally once a day on days 2-5)
- **Tonsillitis**
  - » (500 mg orally once a day for 3 days)
- **Sinusitis**
  - » (500 mg orally once a day for 3 days)
- **Gonorrhea**
  - » (2 g orally once or 1 g orally in combination with a cephalosporin like ceftriaxone)
- **Chlamydia**
  - » (1 g orally once)
- **Syphilis** (early)
  - » (2 g orally as a single dose)

- **Pelvic infections**
  - » (Usually require 500 mg IV once a day for 1 or 2 days, followed by 250 mg orally once a day for 7 days)
- **Whooping cough**
  - » (500 mg orally once on day 1, then 250 mg orally once a day for 4 days)
- **Lyme Disease** (early stages)
  - » (500 mg orally once a day for 7-10 days in those allergic to amoxicillin)

Azithromycin is taken 250 mg or 500 mg once daily for a relatively short course of treatment (usually five days). Alternatively, the dose for day 1 is often a "**loading dose**" that is twice the strength (500 mg) taken at once, with day 2-5 being a single dose daily of 250 mg. Take with or without food (some recommend without).

Pediatric dosing is highly variable depending on the infection, but the most common regimen for children 2 years of age and older is 10 mg/kg (maximum 500 mg) on day 1, followed by 5 mg/kg (maximum 250 mg/dose) orally once a day on days 2- 5.

For acute bacterial sinusitis, azithromycin may be taken once daily for three days. If you are taking the 500 mg dosage and have side effects such as nausea and vomiting, diarrhea, or dizziness, drop down to 250 mg. For gonorrhea, one single dose of 2 grams is considered sufficient.

Azithromycin is not known to cause problems in pregnant patients and can be used by those allergic to Penicillin. It is generally safe to use while breastfeeding, although it should be discontinued if diarrhea or a diaper rash develops.

Azithromycin is acceptable for use in those allergic to penicillin-family drugs.

Levofloxacin

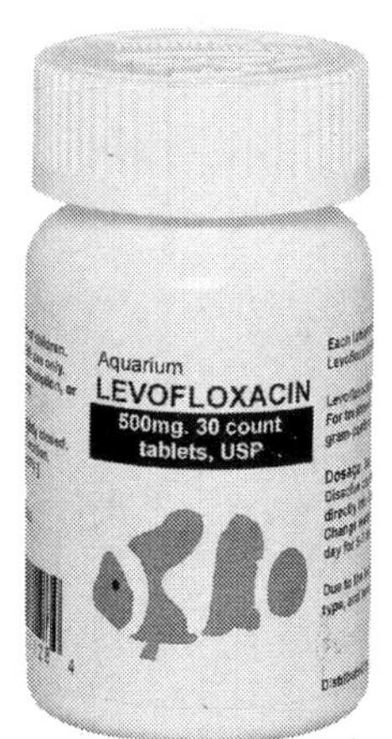

Levofloxacin, like ciprofloxacin, is a member of the fluoroquinolone family. Like other fluoroquinolones, it kills bacteria by inhibiting the reproduction of DNA and bacterial proteins. It comes in 250 mg, 500 mg, and 750 mg dosages. It is considered a relatively simple treatment course, usually requiring one daily dose.

Levofloxacin can be used as a treatment for:

- Pneumonia 500-750 mg orally daily for 7-14 days.
- Bronchitis 500-750 mg orally daily for 7-14 days.
- Sinusitis 500-750 mg orally daily for 7-14 days.
- Skin Infections.
- Prostatitis 500 mg orally daily for 28 days.
- Inhalation and cutaneous anthrax (see below)
- Plague 500 mg orally daily for 10 days.
- Urinary tract Infections 250 mg orally daily for 7 days.
- Chlamydia 500 mg orally daily for 7 days.
- Pelvic Inflammatory Disease (PID) 500 mg daily for 14 days.

Like many antibiotics, there is significant variation in dosing dependent on the infection. For example, a typical course of therapy for respiratory issues might be 500 mg orally every 24 hours for 7 to 14 days or 750 mg orally every 24 hours for 5 days. Doses of 250 mg are often used for urinary infections. For treatment and prevention of Anthrax, the dosage is 500-750 mg orally every 24 hours for 60 days; for prostatitis, it's 500 mg orally every 24 hours for 28 days.

Levofloxacin has not been approved for use during pregnancy. It is, however, acceptable for those allergic to Penicillin. Like ciprofloxacin, negative reactions resulting in severe muscle and tendon damage may occur, as well as other serious effects.

Despite these risks, pediatric use may be considered if older than 6 months of age.

- If less than 50 kg: 8 mg/kg orally every 12 hours, maximum of 250 mg per dose for 10-14 days.
- If at least 50 kg: 500 mg orally 24 hours for 10-14 days.

As with other fluoroquinolones, there are concerns regarding tendon damage and other complications with usage.

Metronidazole

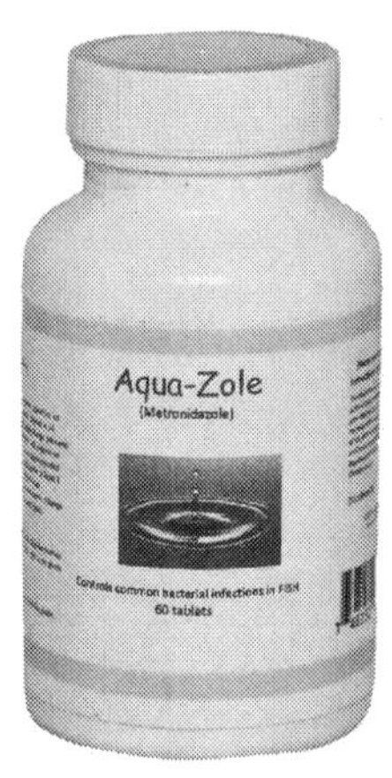

Metronidazole is a bactericidal antibiotic in the nitroimidazole family that is used primarily to treat infections caused by anaerobic bacteria and protozoa. Indeed, the drug is one of the rare examples of an anti-parasitic agent which has also gained broad use as an antibacterial.

Metronidazole works by entering, then blocking, important functions within bacteria and protozoa, resulting in their deaths. Metronidazole is used in the treatment of these bacterial diseases:

- **Diverticulitis (an intestinal infection seen in older individuals)**
  - » (7.5 mg/kg orally every 6 hours for 7-10 days not to exceed 4 g daily; 1 kg = 2.2 pounds)
- **Peritonitis**
  - » (7.5 mg/kg orally every 6 hours for 7-10 days not to exceed 4 g daily)

- **Pneumonias and blood infections caused by** Bacteroides **species**
  - » (7.5 mg/kg orally every 6 hours for 7-10 days not to exceed 4 g daily)
- **Meningitis**
  - » (in IV form)
- **Bone and joint infections**
  - » (7.5 mg/kg orally every 6 hours for 7-10 days not to exceed 4 g daily)
- **Colitis due to Clostridia bacteria** (sometimes from taking antibiotics!)
  - » (500-750 orally every 8 hours for 10-14 days)
- **Bacterial vaginosis**
  - » (500 mg twice daily for 7 days)
- **Pelvic or uterine infections due to STDs, birth issues or miscarriage**
  - » (500 mg orally twice daily for 14 days in combination with other drugs, perhaps doxycycline or azithromycin)
- **Dental infections**
  - » (Metronidazole 400 mg every 8 hours for 5 days; amoxicillin may be added for tooth abscesses or severe disease)
- Helicobacter pylori **infections causing stomach ulcers**
  - » (500-750 mg twice daily for several days in combination with antacids like Omeprazole)

- **Skin and soft tissue infections like cellulitis**
  - » (7.5 mg/kg orally every 6 hours for 7-10 days not to exceed 4 g daily)
- **Wound Infections or following animal or human bites**
  - » (250 to 500 mg orally 3 times a day for 7-10 days or until improved)

And these protozoal infections:

- **Dysentery caused by Entamoeba histolytica**
  - » (750 mg orally 3 times daily for 5-10 days)
- **Intestinal disease caused by Giardiasis**
  - » (250 mg orally three times daily for 5 days)
- Trichomoniasis **(Trich) vaginal infections**
  - » (2 g single dose (4 500 mg tablets at once) or 1 g twice total)

Dosages for metronidazole are highly variable based on the infection that is treated, although you shouldn't ingest more than 4 grams a day. The veterinary equivalent comes in 250 mg and 500 mg. Pediatric dosing is no different. To illustrate, here are the children's dosages and frequency of administration for several infections:

- **Dysentery from** Entamoeba**:** For children, give 35 to 50 mg/kg/day total orally in 3 divided doses for 10 days (no more than adult dosage, of course, regardless of weight).
- **Anaerobic infections (various):** 7.5 mg/kg total orally every 6 hours not to exceed 4 grams daily.
- **Giardia:** For children, give 15 mg/kg/day total orally in 3 divided doses (no more than adult dosage regardless of weight).

Like all antibiotics, metronidazole has a number of side effects and interactions. For example, drinking alcohol while on Metronidazole will very likely make you vomit. Others include diarrhea, nausea, stomach cramps, insomnia and, in some, a metallic taste in their mouth.

Metronidazole should not be used in pregnancy nor breastfeeding, but is acceptable in those allergic to Penicillin.

Ciprofloxacin

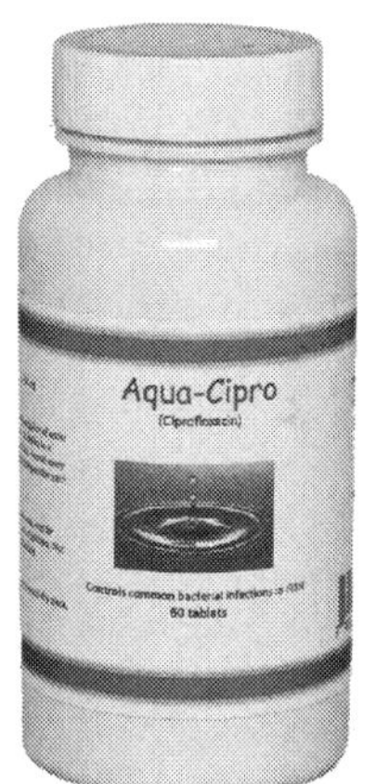

Ciprofloxacin is a bactericidal antibiotic in the fluoroquinolone family. It kills bacteria by inhibiting the reproduction of DNA and bacterial proteins. This drug usually comes in 250 mg and 500 mg doses.

Ciprofloxacin can be used for the following conditions:

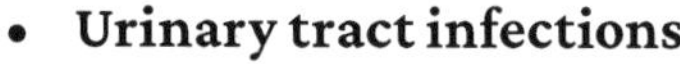

- **Urinary tract infections**
  - » (250-500 mg orally every 12 hours for 7-14 days)
- **Pneumonia, bronchitis, and respiratory infections resistant to other antibiotics**
  - » (500-750 mg orally every 12 hours 7-14 days)
- **Acute sinusitis**
  - » (500 mg orally every 12 hours for 10 days)
- **Skin and soft tissue infections (cellulitis)**
  - » (500-750 mg orally every 12 hours for 7-14 days)
- **Mastitis (even due to MRSA)**
  - » 500 mg every 12 hours for 10-14 days

- **Bone and joint infections caused by bacteria**
  - » (500-750 mg orally every 12 hours for 4-8 weeks)
- **Dysentery and infectious diarrheas** due to *Campylobacter, Shigella*, and *E. coli*
  - » (500 mg orally every 12 hours for 7-10 days)
- **Traveler's Diarrhea prevention**
  - » (500 mg orally once a day for up to 2-3 weeks)
- **Typhoid fever caused by Salmonella**
  - » (500 mg orally every 12 hours for 10 days)
- **Cholera**
  - » (1 g orally once)
- **Inhalational and cutaneous anthrax**
  - » (500 mg orally every 12 hours for 60 days)
- **Plague**
  - » (500-750 mg orally every 12 hours for 14 days)
- **Gonorrhea**
  - » (250 mg one-time dose)
- **Meningitis prevention**
  - » (500 mg orally once)

In most cases, you should give 500 mg twice a day for 7-14 days, with the exception of bone and joint infections (4-6 weeks) and anthrax (60 days). Some milder infections like those affecting the bladder can be treated with 250 mg doses for 3 days. Generally, you would want to continue the medication for 2 days after improvement is noted.

Ciprofloxacin should be taken with 8 ounces of water, with or without food, at the same time each day.

Cipro, while an effective antibiotic, has significant risks due to reports that it can cause weakness in muscles and tendons. Fragile tissues may tear, causing pain, swelling, and joint stiffness, especially in elderly or transplant patients. It is also reported to be responsible for some cases of nerve damage and changes in mental status. Overall, the risks are significant.

Children are also susceptible, so pediatric use is limited to only two conditions: Urinary tract infections caused by *E. Coli* and inhalational anthrax. The pediatric dosage is measured by multiplying 10 mg by the weight in kilograms (1 kg = 2.2 lbs.). The maximum dose should not exceed 400 mg total twice a day, even if the child weighs more than 100 pounds.

Ciprofloxacin has not been approved for use during pregnancy. Although no damage has been documented with breastfeeding, it is rarely used. The drug is acceptable for those allergic to Penicillin.

Ciprofloxacin should be taken with 8 ounces of water, with or without food, at the same time each day.

Fluconazole

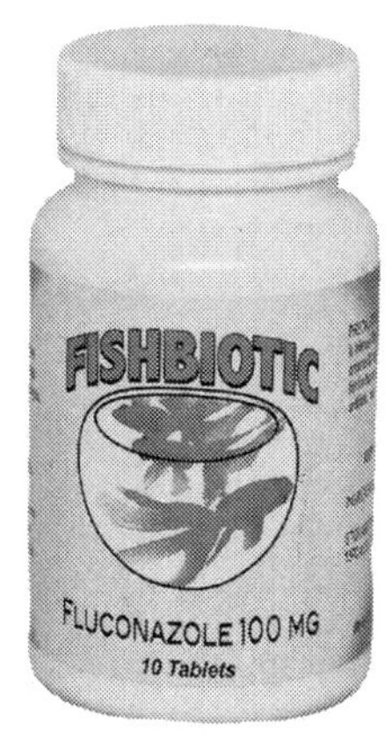

Fungal skin infections most often involve the feet, hands, nails, and scalp. Clotrimazole (Lotrimin) is a good choice as a topical antifungal and doesn't require a prescription. Over the counter miconazole (Monistat) is useful for vaginal yeast infections, but stubborn cases may require an oral anti-fungal like Fluconazole.

Fluconazole, a member of the triazole family, works by interfering with enzymes needed to form the fungal cell membrane. It comes in 50 mg, 100 mg, 150 mg, and 200 mg tablets and oral suspensions. The veterinary equivalent is sold in 100 mg doses.

Fluconazole may be effective in the treatment of a wide range of fungal infections, including:

- **Candidiasis (vaginal)**
  - (150 mg orally as a single dose or, if resistant, 150 mg orally every 72 hours for 3 doses)
- **Oral candidiasis ("Thrush")**
  - (100-200 mg orally once a day for 7-14 days; as oral suspension for infants: 3mg/kg once daily for 7 days)
- **Mastitis due to Candida** (not yet FDA approved)
  - (If clotrimazole or miconazole are ineffective, 200-400 mg loading dose and then 100 to 200 mg once a day for 14 to 21 day; evaluate for signs of bacterial cellulitis mentioned earlier in this book)
- **Onychomycosis (fungal infections of the fingernails or toenails)**
  - (150-300 mg orally once a week for 3-6 months for fingernails or 6-12 months for toenails)
- **Dermatophytosis (ringworm, athlete's foot, jock itch)**
  - (150 mg once weekly for 2-6 weeks)
- **Coccidioidomycosis** (Valley Fever in parts of the Western U.S.)
  - (400-800 mg orally once a day for 3-6 months)
- **Cryptococcosis** (skin, lung, and brain infection caused by an organism found in bird droppings)
  - (400-800 mg orally once a day for at least 8 weeks)
- **Histoplasmosis** (lung infection caused by organisms found in bat and bird droppings; sometimes called "Caver's Disease")
  - (200-800 mg orally once a day for at least 12 months)
- **Pityriasis versicolor** (infection that causes multiple light-colored patches on skin)
  - (50 mg once daily or 150 mg once weekly for 2-6 weeks)

100 to 200 mg of fluconazole orally once a day for 7-14 days is a standard course of treatment for most conditions, although a 150 mg dose taken once may be successful in eliminating vaginal yeast infections. It should be noted that severe cases of fungal infections in internal organs are treated intravenously.

For severe conditions like fungal pneumonia, coccidioidomycosis, cryptococcus, and other serious infections, 400 mg once a day may be required for weeks to months, dependent on the immune status of the patient. For fungal bladder infections, 100-200 mg orally once a day may be effective.

Pediatric dosage ranges from 6-12 mg/kg per day. Duration depends on the disease.

Fluconazole may be taken with or without food. It can be taken even if allergic to penicillin, but not if pregnant. As long as short-term therapy is used, breastfeeding is acceptable.

Common side effects include vomiting, diarrhea, stomach upset, rash, headache, dizziness, and changes in taste sensations. Fluconazole may rarely cause liver dysfunction.

Ketoconazole

Another anti-fungal drug is Ketoconazole. It works by interfering with the formation of the fungal cell membrane.

Ketoconazole is indicated for the treatment of systemic (throughout the body) fungal infections. It is only used for local infections when severe and other anti-fungal medications fail due to the risk of liver malfunction and other adverse effects. In other words, this is not a drug that you'd want to use for a simple toenail fungus.

Ketoconazole is used for:

- **Systemic candidiasis** (same fungus as in vaginal infections)
- **Oral thrush** (mouth infections, usually in infants)
- **Candiduria** (fungus in the urine)
- **Fungal lung infections** (various species)

Identifying fungus in urine, phlegm, or other bodily fluids is relatively simple *if* you have a microscope. Of course, the issues are the cost involved and the need for power to activate the light source.

The oral dose of ketoconazole in adults is 200 to 400 mg daily for two to eight weeks. Nail infections, however, are treated for up to twelve months. The dose in children is usually 50 mg per day for those weighing less than 20 kg and 100mg daily for those 20-40 kg.

Although you might find ketoconazole in veterinary form, other anti-fungal meds have less adverse reactions. Use topical creams or fluconazole unless the situation is dire.

Anti-Viral Drugs

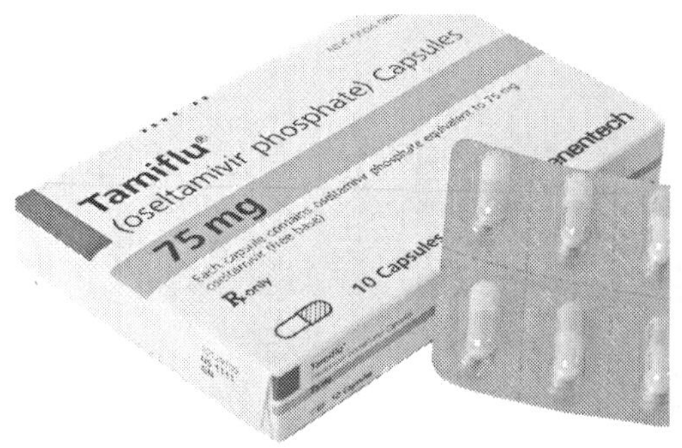

This book is about drugs that kill bacteria. Antibiotics are useless, sadly, against viruses but we feel that a mention should be made about anti-viral drugs. Antiviral drugs would be useful to prevent or treat influenza and treat herpes, chickenpox, and shingles.

One of the most popular anti-viral influenza drugs is called Tamiflu (oseltamivir). Tamiflu gives effective relief against symptoms of influenza and decreases the amount of time your patient would be sick. It can be taken upon exposure to the infection even before symptoms have begun.

If Tamiflu is taken once exposed and before symptoms occur, it might even prevent the illness altogether. This may be a wise strategy if family members are ill with the flu and you haven't gotten it yet.

Taken in the first 48 hours of a flu-like syndrome, Tamiflu may decrease the severity and duration of symptoms. Unfortunately, if taken after this time, it may be less effective. You should know that Tamiflu is specifically meant to treat viral influenza, and won't help much in other viral illnesses, such as Herpes or Ebola.

The adult preventative dose of Tamiflu is 75 mg once daily for 10 days. To treat symptoms, take 75mg twice a day for 5 days. For children, follow the above regimen in the following doses:

- 15 kg (33 lbs.) or less: 30 mg dosage
- 6-23 kg (34-51 lbs.): 45 mg dosage
- 24-40 kg (52-88 lbs.): 60 mg dosage
- Above 40 kg (89 lbs. or more): adult dosage

It should be noted that a one-day treatment is now available comparable to oseltamivir. Known as baloxavir marboxil (Xofluza), it can be used as a one-time dose.

- If patient is under 80 kg: 40 mg orally as a single dose.
- If over or equal to 80 kg: 80 mg orally as a single dose.

Other anti-viral drugs such as Acyclovir or Famciclovir are usually used to treat common herpes-virus related conditions, such as:

Shingles (painful skin eruption)

- Adults: 800 mg every 4 hours for 5 to 10 days
- Children under 40 kg (and older than 2 years): 20 mg/kg 4 times a day for 5 days.

Varicella (chickenpox)

- Adults: 800 mg 4 times a day for 5 days
- Children under 40 kg (and older than 2 years): 20 mg/kg orally 4 times a day for 5 days

Oral/genital Herpes (painful cold or genital sores)

- Adults: 200 mg every 4 hours for 10 days or 400 mg 3 times a day for 7-10 days
- Children under 40 kg (and older than 2 years): 40 to 80 mg/kg a day in 3 to 4 divided doses for 5 to 10 days. Maximum dose should not exceed 1 g per day

PROPER DRUG STORAGE

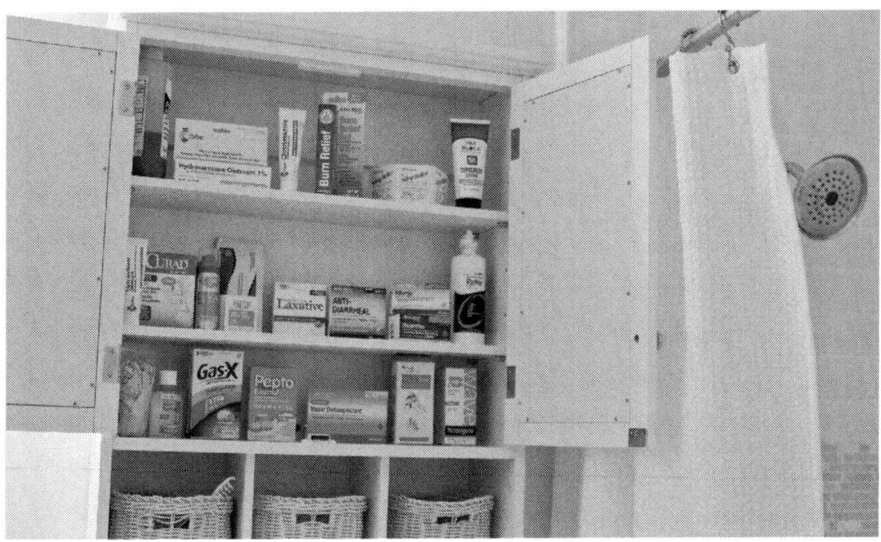

A humid bathroom is a poor location for drug storage

If you find yourself in a remote location or other austere setting, the medicines you've stored may have to stay potent for a long period of time. How medicines are stored can affect their potency over time. To maintain the effectiveness of the drugs, there are several factors that deserve your attention:

Heat: Most medications are meant to be stored at room temperature. Insulin and some antibiotic elixirs are an exception, and should be stored in the refrigerator. A good rule of thumb is that, unless the bottle contains labeling that says otherwise, it's unnecessary (and in many cases, harmful) to freeze or otherwise diverge from the advice given by the manufacturer.

Excessive heat is another factor in losing drug potency. Given the choice, somewhat cooler is probably better than hotter. It's thought that drug effectiveness fades twice as quickly if stored at 90 degrees Fahrenheit than if stored at 50 degrees.

Moisture: Most folks store medications in the bathroom medicine cabinet, but you might be surprised to know that the moisture from showers and baths can degrade the drug significantly. Instead, consider a high shelf in a closet or a dedicated storage box.

Light: Much like excessive exposure to the sun damages skin, light has an ill effect on certain drugs. These meds are commonly stored in brownish-colored bottles. Keep all medicines unopened in their original containers. Once opened, however, it might be a good idea to remove the cotton ball commonly placed with the drug as it could pull moisture into the container.

Many times, it might be hard to tell if a drug has been affected negatively, but some others are pretty obvious. Aspirin pills, for example, can develop a vinegar-like smell (even before the expiration date). Besides smell, a change in color or consistency may signal that a medication has degraded. If pills or capsules are harder or softer than normal or stick together, be wary.

Some people get their meds through the mail. If so, choose overnight shipping whenever possible to avoid prolonged travel time. ABC news reported a 1995 FDA study which found a standard black mailbox can reach 136 degrees in the summer heat. Excessive time in the hot sun or extreme cold for a long period of time causes drug deterioration. A better alternative may be to send them to where you can take possession personally and immediately. For many, this might be their workplace as opposed to their home.

One of the questions we're often asked is whether drugs will benefit from vacuum sealing. Although you'll find opinions everywhere, there doesn't seem to be any conclusive hard data on the issue. We would expect that more drugs would be vacuum packed by the manufacturer if it were that important a factor in maintaining potency. Having said that, pharmaceutical companies want you to discard older meds so they might not be motivated to do so.

Vacuum packing would protect against moisture but wouldn't affect important preservation aspects like temperature or light. As meds do best in their original containers, it seems that (with the possible exception of powder packets) vacuum packing wouldn't be necessary as a storage method.

In the final analysis, storing all meds in cool, dark, dry conditions will give them the longest shelf life possible.

One final bit of advice: It's critically important to be sure that all medications are kept out of the reach of children. Childproof lids are meant to help you achieve this goal, but consider a storage box with a lock as well for an extra layer of security.

EXPIRED DRUGS

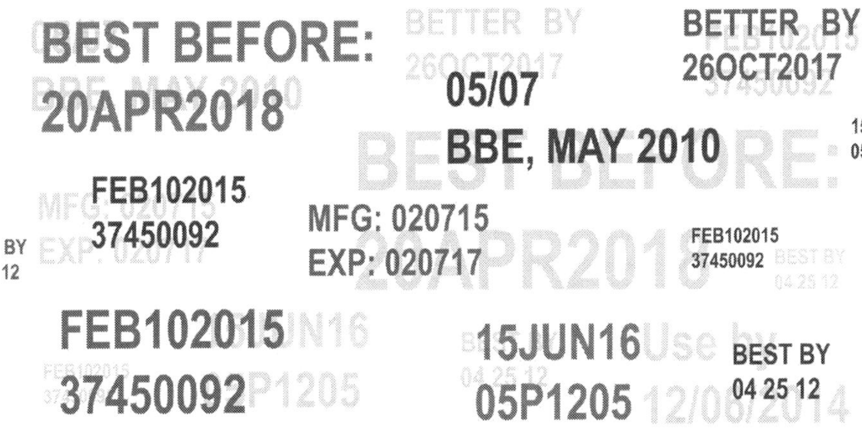

What do expiration dates mean?

Years ago, we wrote an article relating to expiration dates on medications: What they mean, what they don't mean, and what to do in long-term survival scenarios. An online search will find some confusing information that tells you how dangerous expired drugs are; yet, at the same time, the same sources state that if they're all you've got, you should probably use them.

Our focus is medical preparedness for major disasters and long-term survival; having a strategy of putting together stockpiles of supplies that might save a life in times of trouble. In normal times, when you can just call your doctor for a fresh prescription, seek modern care by qualified professionals.

What is an expiration date? Expiration dates were first mandated in the US in 1979. They signify the last day a drug company will guarantee 100% potency of a medicine.

These medicines do not, with few exceptions, turn toxic after the expiration date. If stored properly, the grand majority of expired antibiotics are not dangerous. The expiration date relates to the strength, not the toxicity, of a medication.

In many cases, drugs in pill, powder, or capsule form will be 100% potent for years after their expiration date.

How can we make this statement?

Government agencies like the Department of Defense stockpiles millions of medication doses for use in national disasters. In the past, when those drugs expired, they were simply discarded.

This amounted to tens of millions of dollars wasted, so a study was performed called the "**Shelf-Life Extension Program**." This program evaluated 122 drugs, including some of the antibiotics discussed in this book. The results showed that most medications, as long as they were in pill or capsule form, maintained their potency, sometimes for years after their expiration dates.

These findings led the government to declare "emergency use extensions" of expiration dates for certain drugs as needed. For example, during the 2009 swine flu epidemic, a 5-year extension was given for the anti-viral drug Tamiflu.

As you can imagine, many are reluctant to keep expired meds. Of course, as long as old drugs can be replaced with new ones, this is perfectly reasonable. But if you are the person medically responsible for your family off the grid, you may have to decide one day if a truly major disaster occurs: whether or not to use an expired medication to save a life.

Let's say a loved one is fading from an infection. Something bad has happened and you're off the grid with little or no hope of getting to modern medical care. You have an expired bottle of antibiotics. What are you going to do? Someone you love is dying. Are you going to use the expired drug or not?

Sometimes, the issues facing the family medic in a catastrophe will be very basic. What's the problem? Do I have medicine that can treat it? Could this medicine, although it has expired, possibly save a loved one? If the answer is yes, can you really choose to *not* use it?

Not all drugs keep as well as others. Certain drugs like tetracycline were reported to cause kidney toxicity when expired. This caused considerable concern in the 1960s and 1970s. People, particularly children, developed kidney dysfunction after receiving outdated tetracycline. In these cases, the cause was found to be a degradation product of the medicine called anhydro-4-epitetracycline.

This seems to be less of an issue after a new formulation substituted citric acid for lactose (at least according to a 1991 report from the World Health Organization). Having said that, tetracycline is an old drug; there are newer relatives available for the disaster medicine cabinet. Kidney issues are rare in patients who take doxycycline as long as they start out with normal renal function.

The use of expired medications will continue to be controversial. If it's all you have when modern medicine is not an option, you may have to make some tough decisions. Do your research and come to your own conclusions.

SECTION 5

✚✚✚

ESTABLISHING A "SICK ROOM"

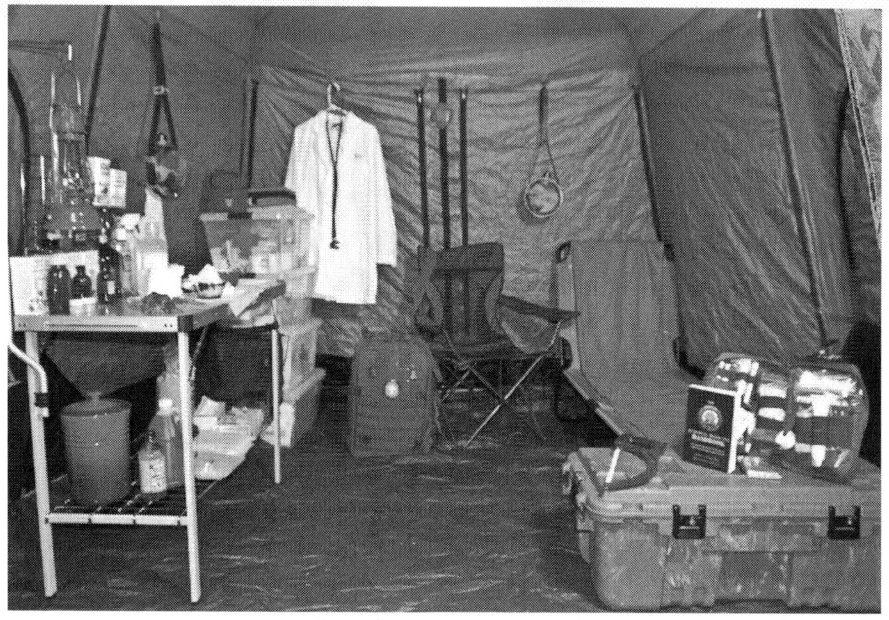

A well-equipped sick room can be put together quite easily

THE EFFECTIVE SICK ROOM

In outbreaks of infectious disease, the challenge for the medic is healing the sick while preventing contagion in the healthy. To succeed, a sick room must be chosen as the place where the infected can rest and recover while not exposing other to the illness. It should be possible to put together a sick room that will minimize the chance of infectious disease running rampant throughout the entire family.

The sick room should be well-lit and have good ventilation. Adequate lighting makes it easier for you to monitor physical signs in your patients. Good air flow in the unit helps decrease the concentration of bacteria and other pathogens in the air. This is important for outbreaks spread by air droplets whether they are bacterial and viral in nature.

A door or other barrier, even if it's just plastic sheeting, is required to separate the sick room from common areas like the kitchen. Dependent on the total space involved, keep the sick room as far away from daily "traffic" as possible. Needless to say, infected individuals should be strictly barred from entering common areas.

Furnishings should be minimal, with a solid work surface, an exam area, and bed spaces. Fabric surfaces, such as you see in sofas, carpets, etc. can harbor pathogens and should be avoided if possible. Even bedding might best be covered in plastic. The more areas that can be disinfected easily, the better.

You must also have a way to eliminate waste products from those that are ill. In most cases, immersion in a container with bleach is sufficient. For extremely contagious diseases, some have suggested incineration.

Here are the items you'll need:

- Disinfectants (household bleach, rubbing alcohol, tincture of Iodine)
- Buckets
- Work table and chair
- Bedding (cotton sheets, etc.)

- Utensils
- Plastic sheeting
- Hand basin with soap, hand sanitizers
- Personal protection gear (discussed next)

A station near the entrance of the room for masks, gloves, gowns, and disinfecting would be very helpful. You'll need a basin with water, soap or other disinfectant, and towels that should be kept for exclusive use by the caregiver. If at all possible, there should only be one person involved in caring for the sick. The less exposure, the less chance of transmitting disease to the rest of the family or group.

One overlooked item that is useful is a noisemaker. Many sick patients are too weak to call out and a noisemaker of some sort will allow you to know when you are needed. It also gives some assurance to the ill that, although you're not always in the room, they are not ignored.

PERSONAL PROTECTION GEAR

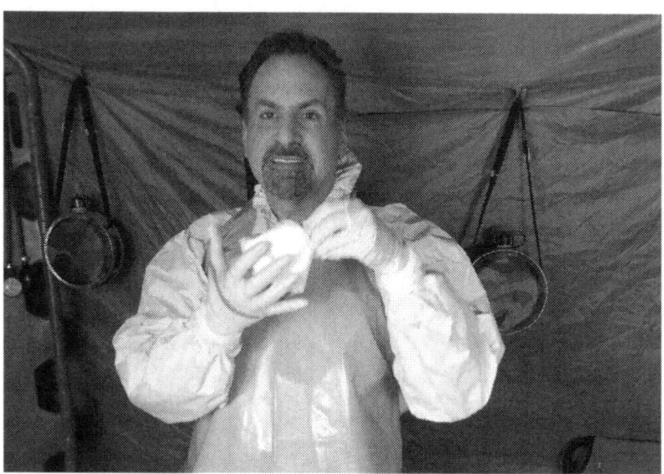

Highly contagious diseases require full- body protection gear

Having knowledge of infectious diseases and how to treat them is very important, but you will be more effective in preventing their spread by having some supplies. Which supplies depend somewhat on the nature of the disease itself and the risk that the healthy population will be exposed to it.

Before you can be effective in healing the sick in an epidemic, you must avoid becoming another of its victims. In a truly virulent outbreak, like the Ebola epidemic of 2014, being a medical worker was one of the principal ways to get (and die of) the disease. As such, strict protocols regarding what items to wear were formulated. In addition, a uniform way to don (put on) and doff (take off) equipment became important in safeguarding the caregivers.

What supplies you should have are separated into two categories: what you should wear and what you should use. First, we'll discuss what armor would give you the most protection. In general order of how you should put them on, you should have:

- Coveralls (with head and shoe covers)
- Masks (N95 or N100)
- Goggles
- Nitrile Gloves
- Duct Tape
- Aprons

About Face Masks

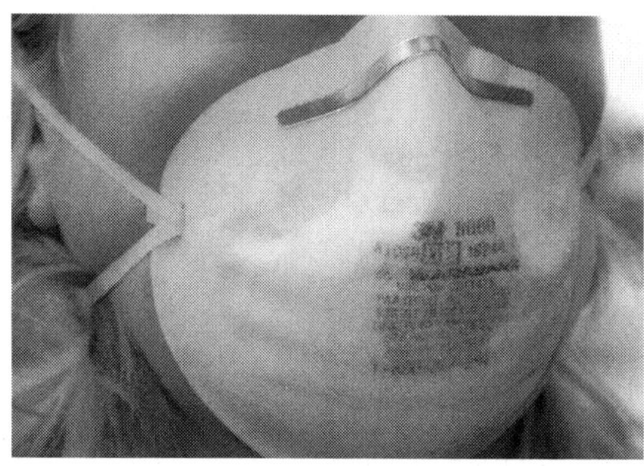

N95 masks are essential supplies for any sick room

Medical masks are evaluated based, partially, on their ability to serve as a barrier to very small particles that might contain bacteria or viruses. These are tested at an air flow rate that approximates human breathing, coughing, and sneezing. As well, masks are tested for their ability to tightly fit the average human face. The most commonly available face masks use ear loops or ties to fix them in place, and are fabricated of "melt-blown" coated fabric (a significant upgrade over woven cotton or gauze).

Standard medical masks have a wide range of protection based on fit and barrier quality; 3-ply masks (the most common version) are more "breathable," as you can imagine, than 6-ply masks. The latter, however, presents more of a barrier.

The upgrade to the basic mask is the N95 respirator mask. N95 Medical Masks are a class of disposable "respirators" that have at least 95% efficiency against particulates larger than 0.3 microns in size. Few people understand just how tiny a micron is. The "N" in N95 stands for non-oil resistant; there are also R95 (oil resistant) and P95 (oil proof) masks, mostly for industrial and agricultural use.

N95 masks protect against many contaminants but are not 100% protective. Although used less frequently due to cost, N99 masks (99%) and N100 masks (99.7%) are also available. Many masks will have a square or round "exhalation valve" in the middle, which helps with breathability.

None of these masks cover the eyes, so it is important to have a mask with a "face shield" or protective eye wear in order to prevent infection.

PUTTING ON AND REMOVING PERSONAL PROTECTION GEAR

Having a supply of personal protection gear is only the beginning. The proper donning of such equipment is imperative if you're going to remain healthy, as is the proper removal. There is a process for safely donning and doffing in a step by step fashion.

It's important to know that every outfit is designed differently, and the process for placement and removal might change depending on the brand of equipment you have. You'll find different recommendations on how to do this, depending on the gear and the department or organization making the recommendation. These are our suggestions. No method is foolproof, however, unless done exactly as described. In any case, you'll don your gear *before* entering the sick room.

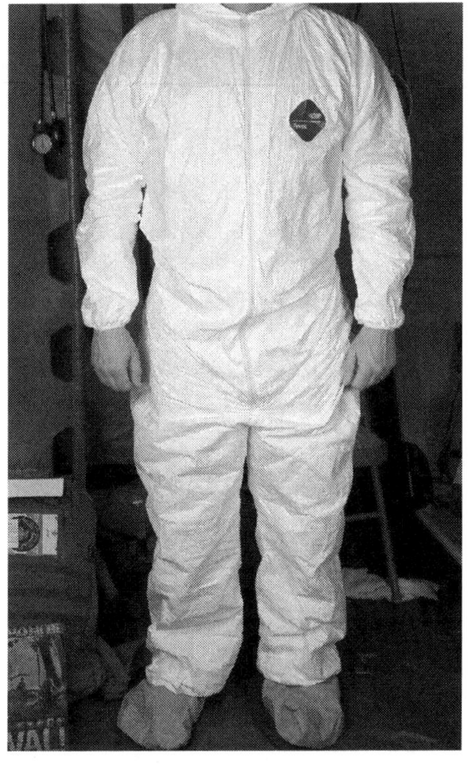

Coveralls zipped up

Donning Your Outfit

First, put on your coveralls but wait to don your hood. If your coveralls don't have a hood, you'll need some type of protective headpiece. If your coveralls have the shoe covers built in, all the better, if they don't, you'll need to place them now. If you have rubber boots, a great item to have in highly contagious settings, put them on now.

Proper Face Mack Placement

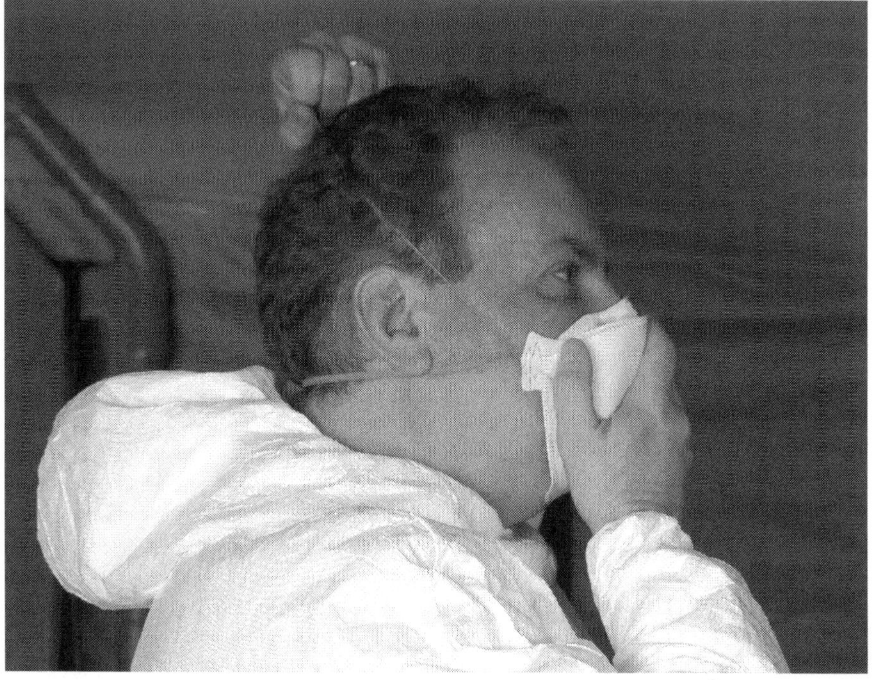

Appropriate placement of face mask

Next, we will put on our mask. A proper seal is necessary to protect your most vulnerable areas like the nose and mouth. You will:

- Expand the mask if it came folded.
- Fit the mask snugly to your face.
- Place the bottom fastening loop so that it is below your ear level, and then the top loop on the back upper part of your head.
- Make a proper seal by pressing the nosepiece of the mask so that it matches your face. You must then test the fit and seal of the mask by breathing in. An indentation should occur in the sides of the masks if the seal is good; air should not escape the outer edges

of the mask when you exhale. Note that facial hair may make it difficult to achieve a solid seal.

- Place protective goggles tightly over your eyes. Some masks come with full face shields built into the item (they may also be separate). Eye protection is important, as blood splatter or aerosol droplets can enter the body through the eyes. Simply using eyeglasses is not effective as a protectant.

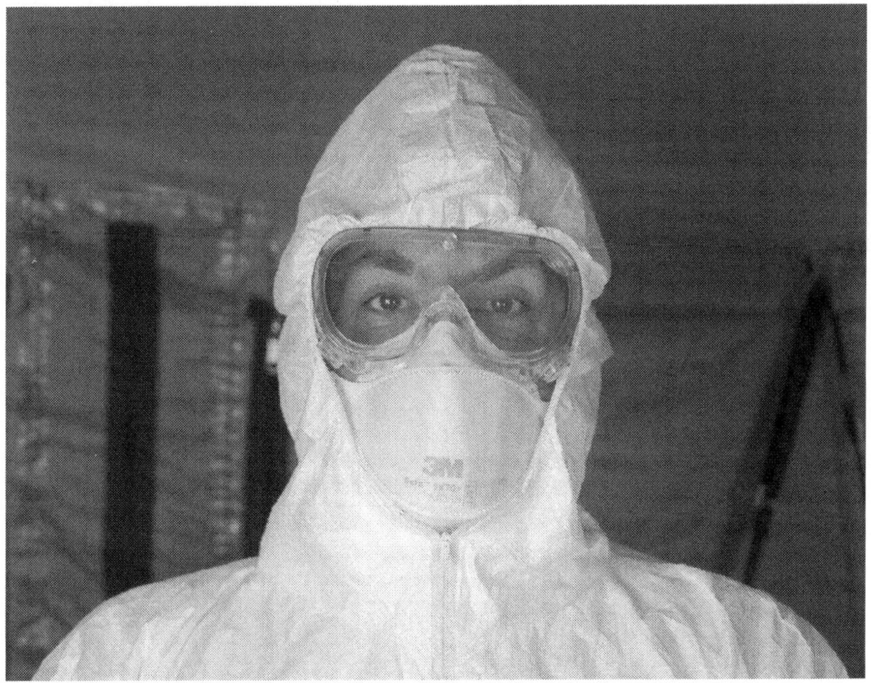

Put hood on

Place the hood over your head. Note that face masks and goggle straps are now protected behind your head. They will be safe to touch during the removal of these items after you're finished caring for the patient. Cover as much of your face as possible.

If there are small exposed areas, perhaps on each cheek, consider placing tape, such as duct tape, to close these defects in your "armor." Full plastic face shields will solve this issue.

Put on two pairs of gloves, one over the other. Most guides will tell you to put on one pair, but we believe there is more protection with two pairs. Be certain to pull the ends of the gloves over your sleeves so that there are no exposed areas.

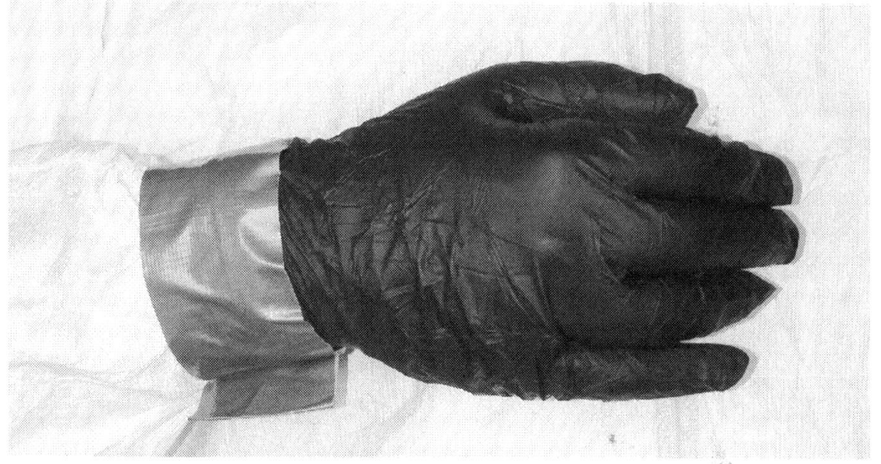

Secure gloves with duct tape

You can tell if you have everything covered simply by stretching your hands over your head. The gloves should still cover the sleeves. Duct tape can be used to secure the wrists of the gloves in place. If taping is necessary, fold over the ends so that you have an easy tab to reach for when you need to remove them.

In contagious disease epidemics, a helper should be present to assure that no mistakes are made and personal protection gear is properly donned.

You will now be ready to deal with a patient that has a highly contagious disease.

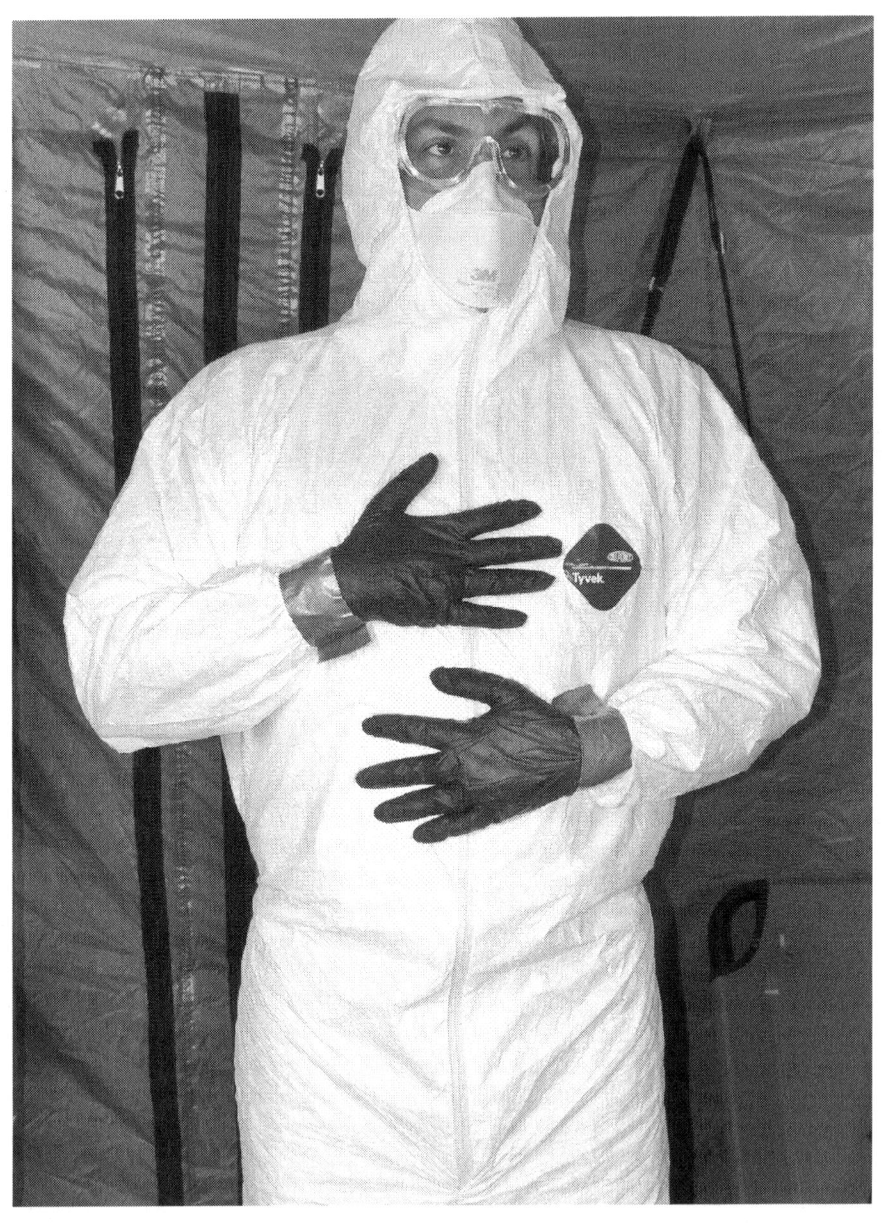
3M
Tyvek

Doffing Your Outfit

The process of removing, or doffing, personal protection gear is just as important as its donning. Leave the patient and go to a designated nearby undressing area or at least get beyond the door of the sick room.

To reduce contagion on your gloves, consider dipping them in disinfectant bleach solution. One part bleach mixed with nine parts water (10% solution) in a large bucket or tub will do. Shake off excess bleach.

Start the process by removing your boots and placing them in the premade tub of disinfectant. Later, you can dry the boots in the sun.

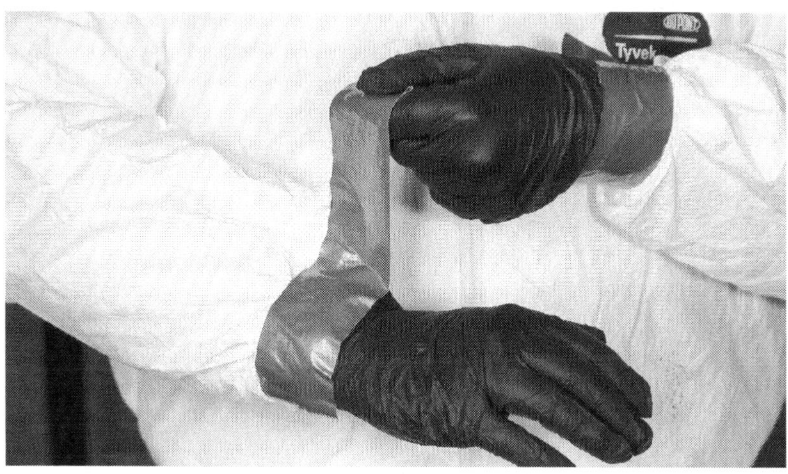

Removing duct tape

- Remove any duct tape you might have on your sleeves or other areas that might prevent you from removing the outfit.
- Remove your outer pair of gloves, which are probably the most contaminated part of your gear. Be careful not to touch your inner pair.

Unless you spent a lot of time facing away from a coughing patient, your outside back is the least dirty. Of course, the inside lining of your gear should still be clean as well. We will use these facts to our advantage in the remainder of our doffing.

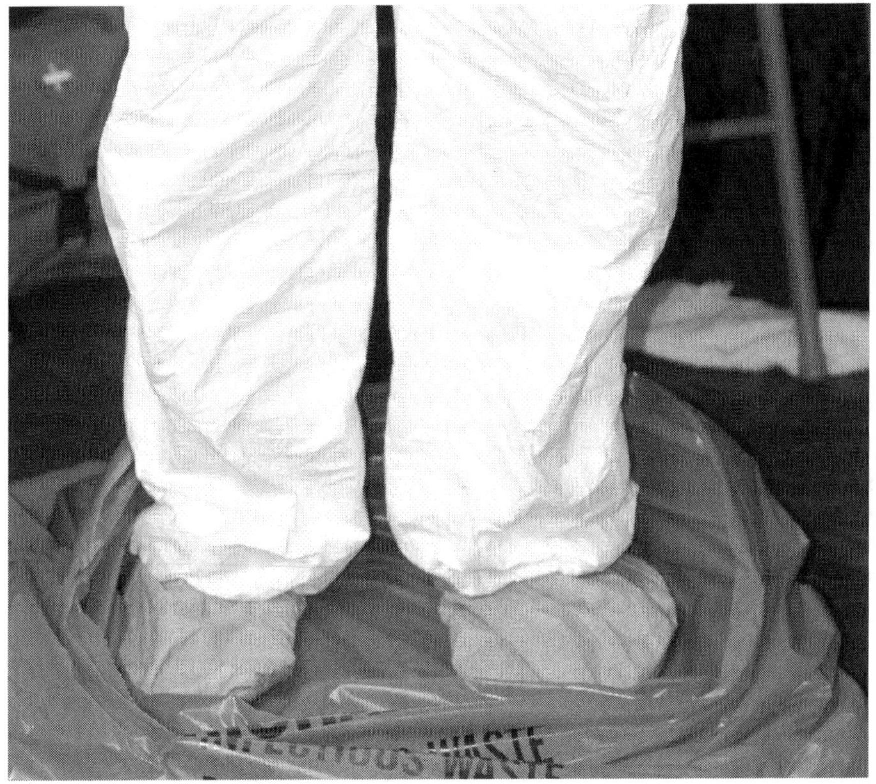

Stand in trash bag and make sure every item goes into it close up

Now you are still wearing your inner pair of, hopefully, clean gloves. Pick up a large hazardous materials bag, open it and place it on the ground. You will do your entire doffing process while standing in this bag.

Evert the edges of the hood inside out so that you can see the inside (clean) lining.

If you are using googles (as opposed to a face mask with shield), remove them by grasping the back of the strap and pulling it over your head. If your goggles are not disposable, place them in a bucket with bleach and water. Keep your mask on.

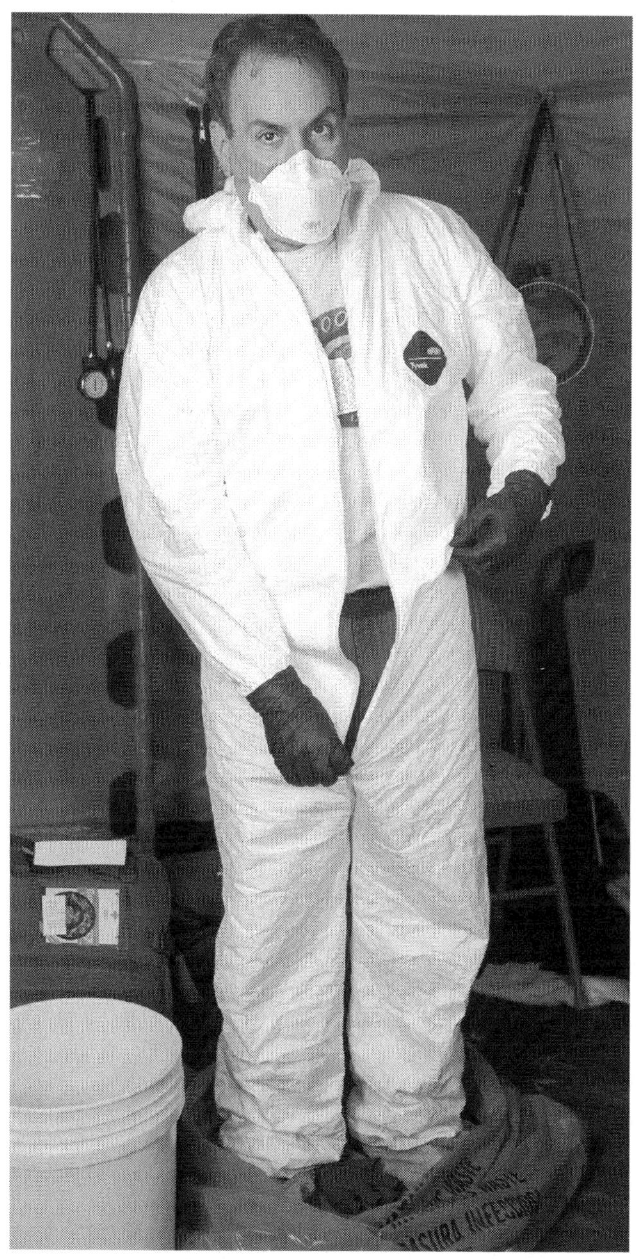

Unzip coveralls and let fall into biohazard bag

Next, unzip your coveralls. By touching the outside of the coverall, your gloves are no longer considered clean at this point; you'll have to be careful to avoid contamination. Some recommend unzipping the coveralls at the beginning, but I think this exposes you to contamination for a longer period of time.

Grab your coveralls with your gloved hand so as to turn it inside out and remove them from one shoulder. Once off the shoulder, use your gloves, now covered by the fabric, to reach behind and pull the coveralls over the other shoulder. Let the coveralls fall to your feet. Avoid touching your clothes with your (contaminated) gloves.

Once the coveralls are at your feet, remove the sleeves so that the gloves are removed along with them in the same motion.

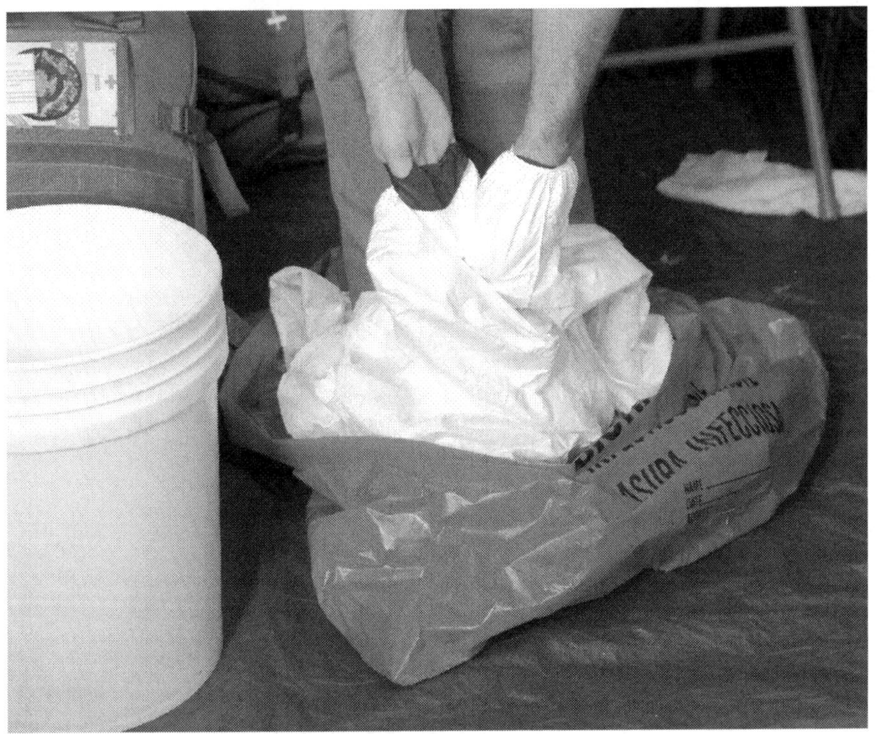

Remove sleeves, before gloves

Once one glove is off, grasp the inside of the other sleeve with your hand, taking care to remove the last glove with its coverall sleeve in one action. Your entire outfit should now be in the hazardous materials bag except for your mask.

Now, without touching the mask itself, lift the loops from behind your head and, then, only holding the loops, drop the mask inside the bag. Step outside the bag before dropping the mask, just in case it hits your pants leg.

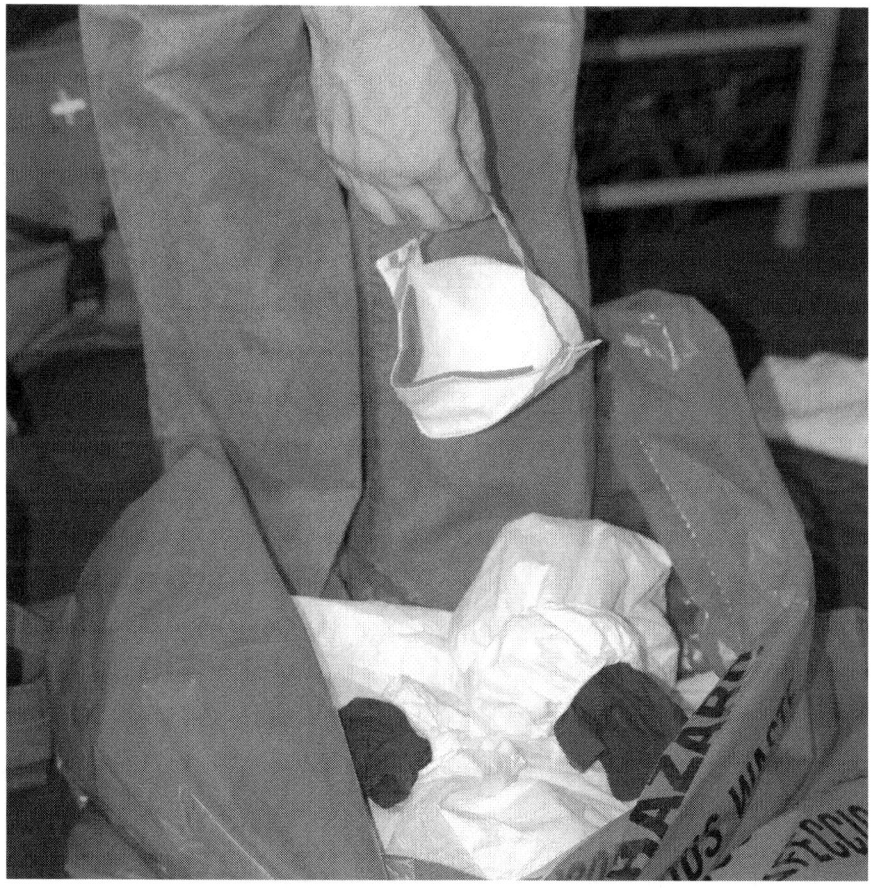

End by dropping mask into biohazard bag

You are now completely undressed and all contaminated materials are in the hazardous waste bag. Allow us to stress that this is just one way that you can safely put on and remove personal protection gear using the items that we recommend. There are variations on this procedure, so do your own research and make your own conclusions. In every case, however, finish by immediately performing rigorous hand washing with soap and water or an alcohol-based sanitizer.

SICK ROOM SUPPLIES

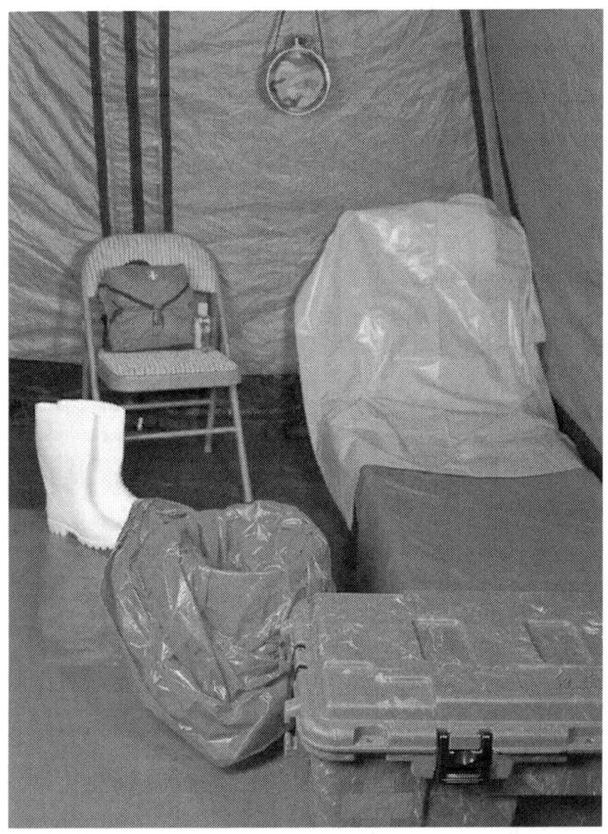

Now that we've discussed what you should wear, here are supplies that you'll want on hand for use in the sick room:

- Hand Sanitizers
- Alcohol, BZK wipes
- Hazardous Waste Bags
- Tissues
- Soap and Water
- Chlorine Bleach (1 part bleach to 9 parts water) solution
- Thermometers

Although this book deals primarily with antibiotics, what other medicines would be useful in an epidemic? The drugs below can treat some of the symptoms you might see in your patient:

- Fever Reducers (acetaminophen)
- Pain Relief (acetaminophen)
- Decongestants (pseudoephedrine, phenylephrine)
- Anti-Diarrheals (loperamide)
- Vitamins and Natural Immune Boosters
- Oral Rehydration Solutions

Making Oral Rehydration Solution

In the Ebola epidemic, many of those who perished simply died of dehydration. You won't have large quantities of IV equipment and fluids, so you will have to make do with oral rehydration. Although commercial solution packets are inexpensive and widely available, you can also make your own using this formula:

- 6-8 level teaspoons of sugar to a liter of clean water
- ½ teaspoon salt per liter (sodium chloride)

- 1/4 teaspoon salt substitute per liter. You'll find in the supermarket where they sell table salt. It's used for people who can't tolerate salt for medical reasons but like the taste of it. This will add potassium chloride to the solution.
- A pinch of baking soda/liter for bicarbonate.
- Double the amount of water in the solution for use in children.

SECTION 6

WOUND CARE

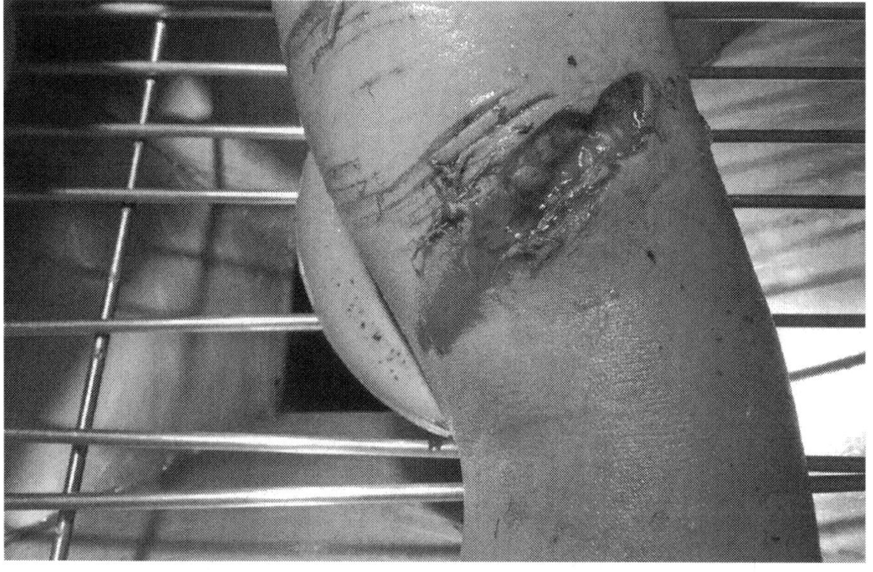

Lacerations are prime areas for infection

WOUND CARE BASICS

Although the sick room will be important to control the spread of epidemic diseases, it will also be a useful treatment room for wound infections. Survival in the aftermath of a major disaster will require the performance of duties to which the average person is not accustomed. These activities may lead to injuries which can become infected. The medic must have a strategy to keep open wounds clean.

Every wound is different and must be evaluated separately. If not present when the wound is incurred, begin by asking the simple question, "What happened?." A look around at the site of the accident will give you an idea of what type of debris you might find in the wound and the likelihood of infection Always assume a wound is dirty initially.

The physical examination of a wound requires the following assessment: Location on the body, length, depth, and the type of tissue involved.

If the injury breaches the **dermis**, we refer to it as a laceration and is more serious. In cases where a flap of tissue has been traumatically removed, it is known as an **avulsion**. In most areas of the body, below the dermis you will find a layer of subcutaneous fat; below that, muscle and connective tissue (also known as fascia) and, finally, bone.

Once the skin is entered, infection can easily follow. A wound that extends more deeply will require a close look to see what layers have been damaged. Subcutaneous fat will appear yellow, and muscle will appear a dark red (think steak). Connective tissue is usually grayish white.

Once below the level of the skin, larger blood vessels and nerves may be involved. Assess circulation, sensation, and the ability to move the injured area. You will notice more problems with vessel and nerve damage in deep lacerations and crush injuries.

For an extremity injury, evaluate what we call the "Capillary Refill Time" to test for circulation. To do this, press the nail bed or finger/toe pad; in a person with normal circulation, this area will turn white when you release pressure and then return to a normal color within 2 seconds. If it takes longer or the fingertips are blue, you may have a person who has damaged a blood vessel.

If motor function or sensation is decreased (test by lightly pricking with a safety pin beyond the level of the wound), there may be nerve damage. These are signals that your patient will require acute care as soon as possible.

Care For Wounds At Risk For Infection

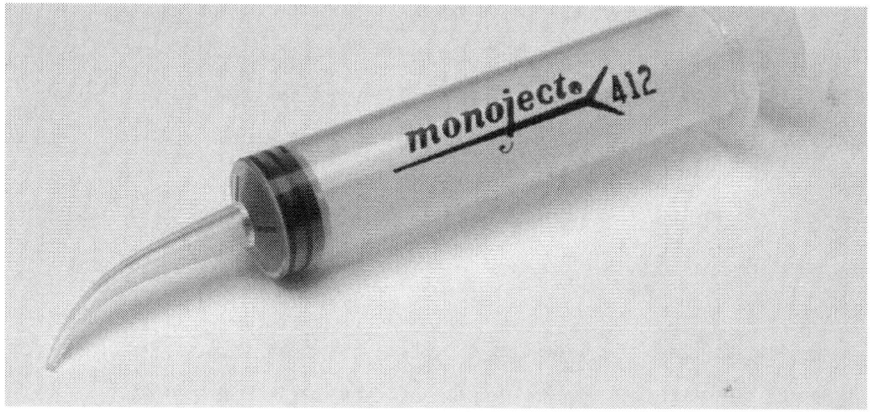

A 60 t0 100 cc syringe will work well to irrigate an open wound

In order to fully assess an open wound and prevent infection, it is important to clean the wound area thoroughly. Inflammation, infection, or residual debris may delay (or even prevent) adequate healing.

Antiseptic solutions such as betadine (povidone-iodine) solution may be helpful if very dilute, but studies have shown that water that is safe to drink is just as good for **irrigation** purposes. If the irrigation solution is not at least of that quality, bacteria might be introduced into even the cleanest wound.

Hydrogen Peroxide or alcohol has been put forth as options to clean an open wound. These substances may kill bacteria but, unfortunately, also harm traumatized tissue, slowing the healing process.

With regards to wound care, the most dangerous source of contamination may be the hands of the caregiver. For this reason, a good supply of gloves is needed to protect the patient and the provider. Nitrile gloves have replaced latex due to the epidemic of latex allergies seen in the recent past.

Effective irrigation applies strong water pressure when cleaning the wound. Using a 60cc syringe to achieve this pressure will cause bacteria adherent to the tissues to dislodge. All wound surfaces should be irrigated; pull the wound edges open if necessary to reach the deepest layers. Repeat this procedure and re-examine for remaining debris until clean.

If no syringe is available, wipe with a wet, clean compress using gauze or cloth. Keeping the area moist will help rehydrate the wound and improve healing. Many recommend a plastic bag with a pinhole in it to irrigate a wound, but it is questionable whether you can achieve an appropriate pressure (about 12 PSI) using this method. Your goal is to flush out all the debris that may be both a focal point for infection and contain toxins that further damage the tissue.

Lacerations are often closed with sutures, staples, or glues but this is very risky with a contaminated wound. Take the example of the young woman in Georgia that was injured in a zipline accident: Her wound was closed with 22 staples at the local hospital. Shortly thereafter, an infection (necrotizing fasciitis) developed in the deep tissues that eventually required amputation.

The time period from injury to wound evaluation is important if you have the skill to close a wound. No more than eight hours is considered appropriate for laceration repair (perhaps a little longer for the face and scalp). Lean towards keeping the wound open if there is a chance you can get your patient to a modern medical facility.

If you choose to close the wound with sutures or staples, cover it with antibiotic topical ointment. This is not appropriate with glues, however; the glue is degraded by the ointment and the closure may fall apart. Often, special closure strips like Steri-Strips with tincture of benzoin will be all that is needed.

OPEN WOUND CARE

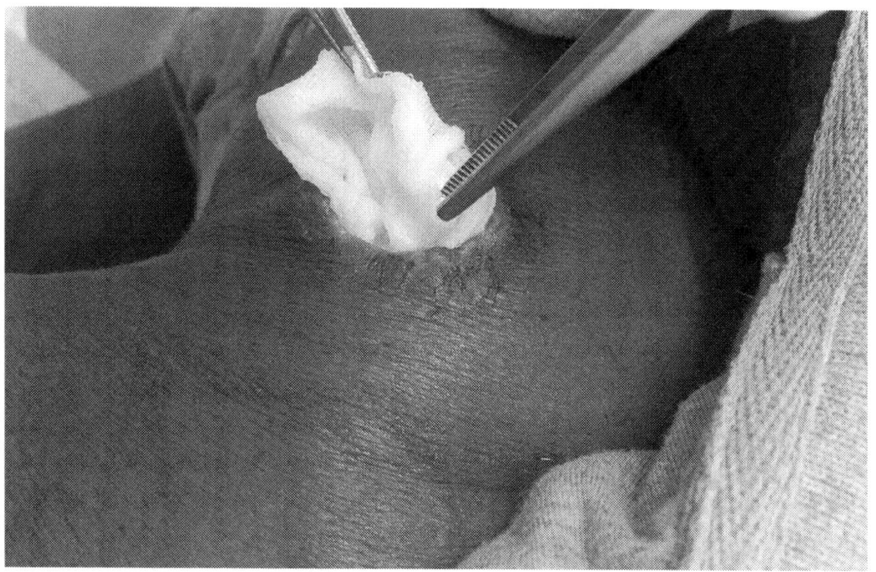

Pack an open wound at least twice a day

Healing occurs in most cases of open wounds as long as the wound is kept moist and clean. This type of healing is known as "**granulation**" or "**secondary intention**."

Once you have aggressively cleaned and irrigated the wound to remove dead tissue and debris, apply a moist, sterile dressing to the open wound directly and up to the level of the skin. The wound is then covered with a dry dressing and tape. This is known as a "wet-to-dry" dressing.

A moist healing environment will help prevent cell dehydration and promote the development of better circulation in the wound. Moisture also reduces pain and leads to a better cosmetic result.

An antibiotic cream may be useful on the skin edges to promote healing while the wound is healing. A natural alternative is raw, unprocessed honey.

Dressing changes should be done at least daily (twice a day is better) until the injured party is able to access professional care or the wound has granulated completely.

Each time a dressing is changed, irrigate with sterile water or saline solution and note the status of the tissues. Infection can often be seen on the skin edges in the form of redness, swelling, and heat. This is known as "**cellulitis**" (discussed earlier) and may progress to an infection to the entire

The decision to use antibiotics should be made early, usually within 3-6 hours after the injury was incurred. The deeper the injury, the more you should lean towards starting therapy. Wounds that are most likely to be infected are animal bites or those lacerations contaminated with feces, saliva, or other bodily secretions.

Here are some suggestions for supplies you should have if you will be responsible for wound care:

- Sterile gauze dressings (these come in various shapes and sizes; have a good quantity and variety in your kit)
- Antiseptic solution/wipes (alcohol, BZK, Betadine)
- Water purification tablets
- 60cc or 100cc irrigation syringe
- Nitrile gloves
- Triple antibiotic ointment
- Ibuprofen (Advil) or Acetaminophen (Tylenol) and other OTC meds
- EMT shears (bandage scissors)—to cut clothes away for better visualization of the wound.
- Adhesive Bandages (Band-Aids or, alternatively, Second Skin)
- Paper or cloth medical tape (Duct tape will do in a pinch)
- Solar blanket (victims of injuries are often in shock and lose heat rapidly)
- Antibiotics

- Splint material for immobilization of an injury (SAM and other splints come in a 36 inch roll you can cut to fit your needs)

A comprehensive list of medical supplies is discussed towards the end of this book.

DAKIN'S SOLUTION

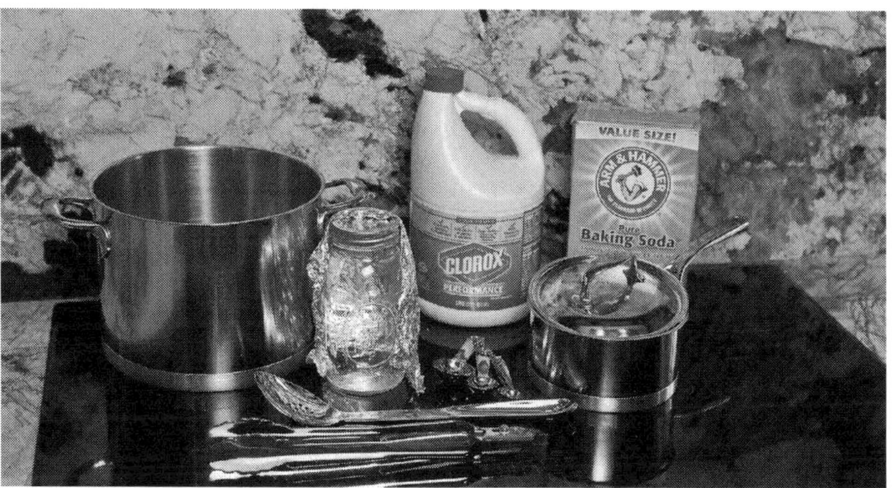

One of the challenges facing the caregiver in austere settings is how to prevent infection in open wounds. A simple and affordable method that was used as far back as World War I may be the answer for the medic: Dakin's antiseptic solution.

Dakin's solution is the product of the efforts of an English chemist, Henry Drysdale Dakin, and a French surgeon named Alexis Carrel. In their search for a useful antiseptic to save the lives of wounded soldiers during WWI, they used sodium hypochlorite (household bleach) and baking soda to make a solution that had significant protective effect against infection. The chlorine in the solution prevented the accumulation of bacteria in open wounds.

(Historical aside: At the same time, both sides in the war were also using chlorine in gaseous form as an anti-personnel weapon!)

As an antiseptic for austere wound care, Dakin's is especially useful for its activity against viruses, fungi, and problem pathogens like MRSA.

Today, Dakin's solution is still considered by many practitioners to be effective enough for use after surgery and on chronic wounds like bedsores. It's easily prepared and can be made stronger or milder by varying the amount of bleach used. Use it in austere settings to clean the wound during dressing changes or to moisten the dressings themselves.

Dakin's Solution Recipe

To make Dakin's solution, you'll need just a few items. This recipe is from Ohio State University's Department of Inpatient Nursing:

- Unscented household bleach (sodium hypochlorite solution 5.25%, avoid more concentrated versions).
- Baking soda (sodium bicarbonate)
- A pan with a lid
- Sterile measuring cup and spoon (sterilize by boiling)
- Sterile canning jar and lid

Of course, wash your hands beforehand, just as you would with any medical procedure. Then:

3) Put 4 cups (32 ounces) of water into the pan and cover with the lid.
4) Boil the water for 15 minutes with the lid on.
5) Remove from the heat source.
6) Use the sterile spoon to add ½ teaspoon of baking soda to the water.
7) Add bleach (sodium hypochlorite 5.25%) in the amount needed (see below).
8) Pour into sterile canning jar and close with a sterile lid.
9) Label and store in a dark place.

The amount of sodium hypochlorite to add depends on whether the wound is infected and how severely:

- Full strength (0.5%): 95 ml (about 3 oz. or 6 tablespoons)
- Half strength (0.25%): 48 ml (3 tablespoons plus ½ teaspoon)
- 1/4 strength (0.125%): 24 ml (1 tablespoon plus 2 teaspoons)
- 1/8 strength (0.0625%): 12 ml (2 ½ teaspoons)

Note: 3 teaspoons = 1 tablespoon = 14.7 ml; 2 tablespoons = 1 US ounce = 29.5 ml

Lower strengths are appropriate for regular preventive wound care, while the higher concentrations may help treat wounds that are currently infected.

Once canned, it's said that Dakin's solution will remain potent for about 30 days. Store in a dark location or cover well for the best longevity. For use in austere settings, however, make it as needed for wounds or maybe just produce a few jars at a time. Once a jar is opened, discard the remainder after a day or so.

You may also consider Century Pharmaceutical's buffered version of Dakin's. The company states that they have tested their solutions and found unopened bottle shelf life to be 12-24 months. They also claim that opened bottles are good for 2-3 months if "kept free of contamination," stored at room temperature, and protected from light.

Using Dakin's Solution on Wounds

Pour into wound once daily for mildly infected wounds, twice daily for heavily infected wounds with drainage of pus. Alternatively, moisten (not soak) dressings used inside the wound (not on top of the skin) with a mild strength solution and observe progress.

Given the fragility of newly-formed cells in a healing wound, we would prefer using it as a cleansing agent as opposed to a component of a wet dressing. Having said that, if you're dealing with a severe infection (as opposed to preventing one), it may be reasonable to incorporate Dakin's into the dressing.

1/8 strength (or less) Dakin's solution can be used as a mouthwash for infections inside the oral cavity, but must *never* be swallowed. Swish for about a minute before spitting it out no more than twice a week.

Full strength Dakin's solution may irritate skin, so consider protecting skin edges with petroleum jelly or other skin protectant/moisture barrier. Look for evidence of skin rashes, burning, itching, hives, or blisters. If irritation occurs, drop down to a milder strength or discontinue. Do not use in those allergic to chlorine.

Sterile Saline Formula

It should be noted that not all practitioners agree about the benefits of Dakin's solution. Certainly, there may be other options with regards to regular wound care, including sterile normal saline and sterilized tap water. Although some physicians consider Dakin's solution controversial, nearly all medical professionals are comfortable with sterile saline when it comes to long-term wound care.

To make Sterile Saline Solution, follow this recipe:

- Place one liter of water into a pot.
- Add two teaspoons of salt.
- Cover with a lid.
- Bring the solution to a boil for one minute (3 minutes at elevations about 6000 feet).
- Let cool with the lid on.
- Use immediately or place in sterile canning jar with a sterile lid.

Either Dakin's solution or sterile saline is well tolerated by patients and simple to make with affordable ingredients. It's another tool in the woodshed for scenarios where modern medical help is not on the way.

RULES FOR PREVENTION OF INFECTION

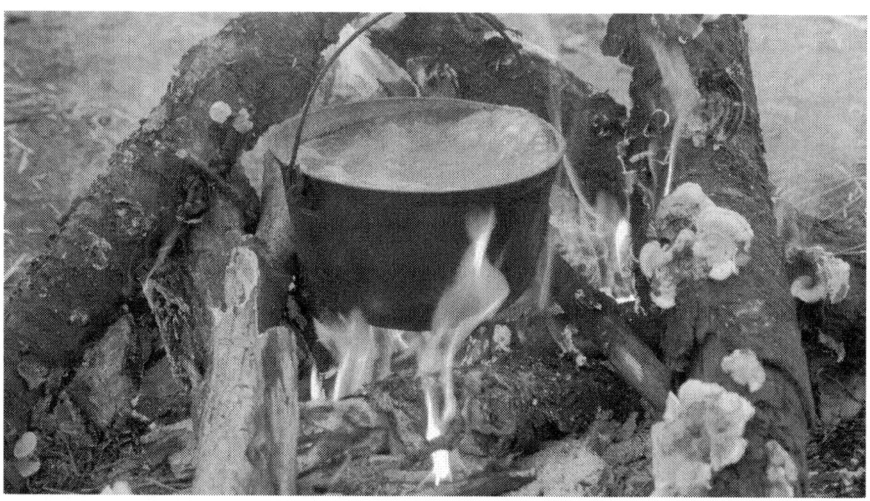

Water can be disinfected by boiling, bleach, iodine, or ultraviolet radiation

Earlier in this book, we described the many ways that infections are spread. We also emphasized the importance of clean water and propeıly prepared food. Purification of questionable water and appropriate cooking methods will save more lives by preventing infection than any antibiotic.

Disinfecting Water

There are several ways to disinfect water:

Boiling: The CDC recommends using a heat source to get your water to a rolling boil for at least 1 minute at sea level and 3 minutes at 2000 meters (about 6560 feet). Alternatively, older methods suggested adding 1 minute per 1000 feet to your boiling time. There are bacteria that may survive high heat, but they are in the minority. Using a pressure cooker would be even more thorough.

Chlorine: Bleach has an excellent track record of eliminating bacteria in water. 12 drops (more with cloudy water) in a gallon of water will do the trick. If you're used to drinking city-treated water, you probably won't notice any difference in taste. Always be certain to wait at least 30 minutes for the chlorine to work its magic.

It should be noted that the pathogen cryptosporidium, mentioned earlier in this book, is relatively resistant and may take days to eliminate. Most other organisms, like *E. coli,* are destroyed in a matter of minutes. If you suspect crypto as the pathogen, boil as described above.

2% Tincture of Iodine: About 16 drops (more if cloudy) per gallon of water will be effective. Wait 30 minutes before drinking.

Ultraviolet Radiation: Sunlight will, indeed, kill bacteria. 6-8 hours in direct sunlight (even better on a reflective surface) will kill most microbes. Fill a clear gallon bottle and shake vigorously for 20 seconds. The oxygen released from the water molecules will help the process along and even improves the taste. Commercial products such as the "Steri-Pen" use ultraviolet light to achieve the same result.

We should emphasize that these methods kill pathogens but don't remove particulates in the water. Filters like the "LifeStraw" or the "Mini-Sawyer" are compact, lightweight, and effective. Filters can also be improvised with a clear 2-gallon bottle and several layers of different-size sand or gravel (some add activated charcoal or food-grade diatomaceous earth).

Food Preparation

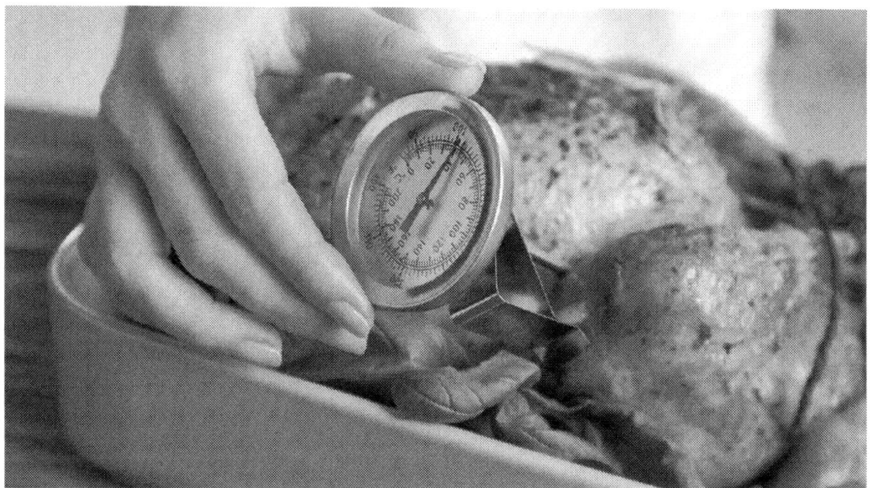

Properly cooking food will greatly decrease the chance for infection

Anyone who has eaten food that has been left out for too long has probably regretted it. The restaurant industry's official line is that it takes about four hours in the open to become contaminated. Food in lemon juice, vinegar or oil may last a bit longer due to the acidic environment or lack of oxygen for bacteria to grow. Despite this, there are **anaerobic** organisms such as the bacteria that causes botulism don't need oxygen to survive.

Food preparation surfaces must be cleaned and dry completely to prevent infection. Your hands, by the way, are a food preparation surface. Wash them thoroughly prior to preparing food. Other surfaces like counter tops, cutting boards, dishes, and utensils should be cleaned with hot water and soap before using them. Soap may not kill all germs, but it helps dislodge them from surfaces. A solution of one part chlorine bleach and nine parts water is an acceptable alternative.

If you have a good supply, use paper towels to clean surfaces. Kitchen towels, especially if kept damp, accumulate a great deal of bacteria. If you are in a truly austere setting where paper towels aren't available, boil cloth cleaning materials before and after use.

Always wash fruits and vegetables under running water before eating them. You're not protected if the fruit has a rind; pathogens on the rind can get on your hand and be transferred to the fruit once you peel it.

Raw meats are notorious for having their juices contaminate food. Prepare meats separately from your fruits and vegetables. A useful item to be certain that meats are safe is a meat thermometer. Indeed, it should be considered a medical supply item. Assuring that meats are fully cooked and reach a consistently appropriate temperature will greatly decrease the chance of "food poisoning."

The safe temperature varies by the type of meat:

- Beef: 145 degrees F
- Pork: 150 degrees F
- Lamb: 160 degrees F
- Poultry: 165 degrees F
- Ground Meats: 160 degrees F
- Sauces and Gravy: 165 degrees F
- Soups with Meat: 165 degrees F
- Fish: 145 degrees F

Additional Recommendations

Once a number of cases of an infectious disease crop up in a community, there will be mention of it in the news. We have all read of some food item that has been recalled due to contamination with bacteria or other pathogen. The same will happen in the early stages of an epidemic.

Besides assuring sanitary practices with regards to drinking water and food preparation, the most important way to prevent the spread of infection is to have a high index of suspicion; that is, to monitor your family closely for those who may develop fever or other signs and symptoms. People are usually most contagious early in the disease process.

Hopefully, you have accumulated the supplies mentioned above and chosen the room or tent that will serve as your "hospital ward." With a predetermined plan of action, setting up an area for infected patients should be relatively easy.

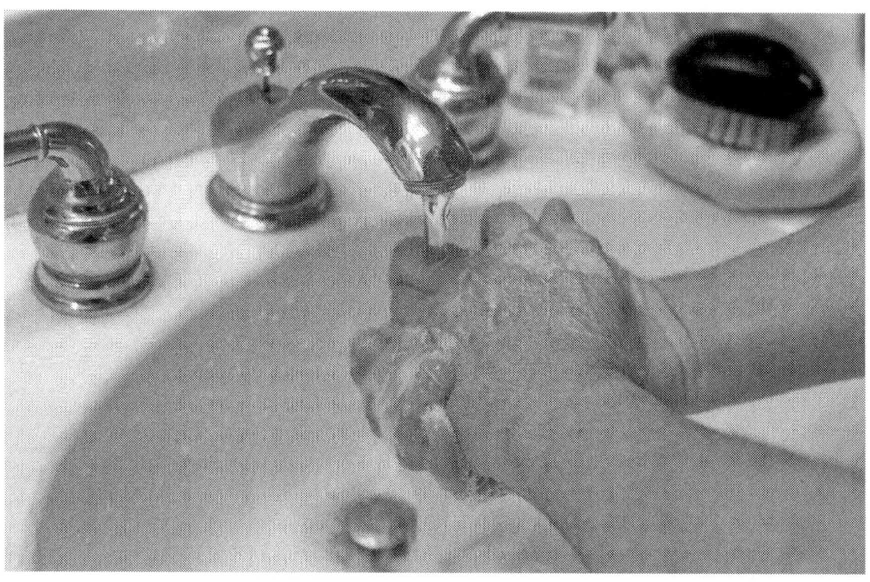

Frequent hand washing is perhaps the most important strategy to prevent infection

To prevent your family from becoming victims of the next epidemic, some simple rules should be strictly enforced. Here are recommendations similar to those put forth by both the Centers for Disease Control and Prevention and the World Health Organization:

- o Wash your hands often with soap and water., alcohol hand sanitizers, or other disinfectant.
- o Avoid touching your mouth, nose, or eyes with your hands.
- o When you cough or sneeze, cover your mouth and nose with a tissue. Then, throw the tissue in the trash. If no tissues are available, cough or sneeze into your sleeve or upper arm, not your hand.
- o Avoid close contact (within 6 feet) with infected individuals without appropriate personal protection gear (this includes "visitors").
- o If multiple individuals are infected, separate them by at least one meter (World Health Organization recommendation)
- o Have separate bedding and utensils for sick individuals.
- o Have a strategy for the safe disposal of waste from infected patients.
- o Place non-infected people requiring medical care in a separate area from those who might be contagious.
- o Place patients with the same infectious disease together (called "**cohorting**").

In epidemic settings, avoid unnecessary trips to areas where the outbreak is active. If this is unavoidable, make sure to:

- Avoid crowded places or buildings where infected patients are housed.
- Wear a face mask if you must go into a crowded area or be within 6 feet of others.
- Consider personal protection gear if you must come into close contact with an infected person, even if outside the sick room.
- Do not, if at all possible, transport infected individuals elsewhere. If there is no choice, keep all windows open.
- If transport is required, disinfect the interior of vehicles after use.

WHAT ELSE DO I NEED TO KNOW?

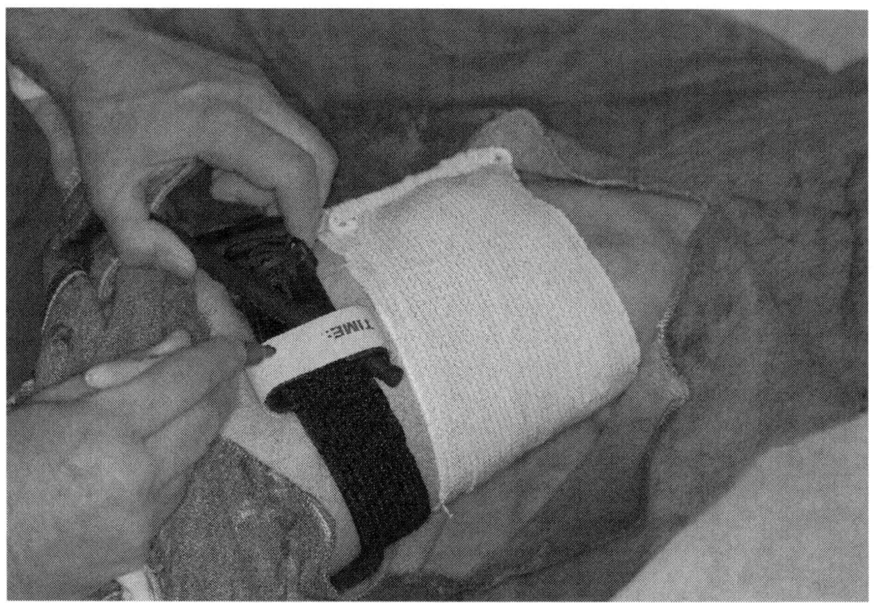

Always place the time of placement so that it is clearly visible

If you have absorbed the information provided in this book, you have gone a long way towards becoming an effective medic with regards to infectious disease diagnosis and care. Hopefully, it has whetted your appetite to learn and put together more supplies that will serve as tools to keep people healthy in times of trouble.

A very reasonable question for an aspiring medic to ask is "What exactly do I need to know?" The answer is: As much as you're willing to learn. You can expect to deal with lots of ankle sprains, colds, cuts, rashes, and other common medical issues that affect people in normal times. In addition, you will need to know how to deal with more significant problems, such as a leg fracture or a bleeding wound. You'll also need to know what medical supplies will be required for more than just infections.

Here are the skills and knowledge that an effective medic would obtain in advance of being thrust into the role of sole caregiver in an austere setting:

- How to take vital signs, such as pulses, respiration rates and blood pressures.
- How to place bandages on injuries.
- How to clean an open wound.
- How to treat varying degrees of burns.
- How to perform a normal delivery of a baby and placenta.
- How to splint, pad and wrap a sprain, dislocation, or fracture.
- How to identify bacterial infectious diseases (such as Strep throat, etc.).
- How to identify viral infectious diseases (such as influenza, etc.).
- How to identify parasitic/protozoal infectious diseases (such as Giardia, etc.).
- How to identify and treat head, pubic, and body lice, as well as bed bug and tick bites.
- How to identify venomous snakes and treat the effects of their bites and those of other animals.
- How to identify and treat various causes of abdominal, pelvic, and chest pain.
- How to treat allergic reactions and anaphylactic shock.
- How to identify and treat sexually transmitted diseases.
- How to evaluate and treat dental problems (replace fillings, treat abscesses, and perform extractions).
- How to identify and treat skin disease and rashes.
- How to care for the bedridden patient (treating bedsores, transport considerations).
- How to teach basic hygiene, nutrition and sanitary practices (this couldn't be more important).

- How to counsel the depressed or anxious patient (you will see a lot of this in times of trouble).
- How to insert an IV (EMT classes teach this).
- How and, more importantly, when to close a wound with sutures, staples, glues, or butterfly closures.
- How to identify the indications for use of different medications (not just antibiotics), essential oils and alternative therapies. As well, know the dosages, frequency of administration, and side effects of those substances.

That's a lot of "how to's," but perhaps the most important skill to obtain is how to *prevent* injuries and illnesses. Simple things, such as assuring your people are appropriately dressed for the weather, will prevent heat stroke and hypothermia. Requiring hand and eye protection during work sessions will prevent injuries. Recognize situations that place your family at risk and you'll avoid many problems.

This is a lot of information to absorb. Don't feel that you can't be of benefit if you only learn some of the above. The important thing is to learn enough to treat some of the more common medical issues.

Once you've learned the basics, you'll be able to take care of 90% of the problems that are brought before you in times of trouble. After that, any additional information you learn will just make you even more effective as a medical resource.

SECTION 7

✚✚✚

MEDICAL SUPPLIES

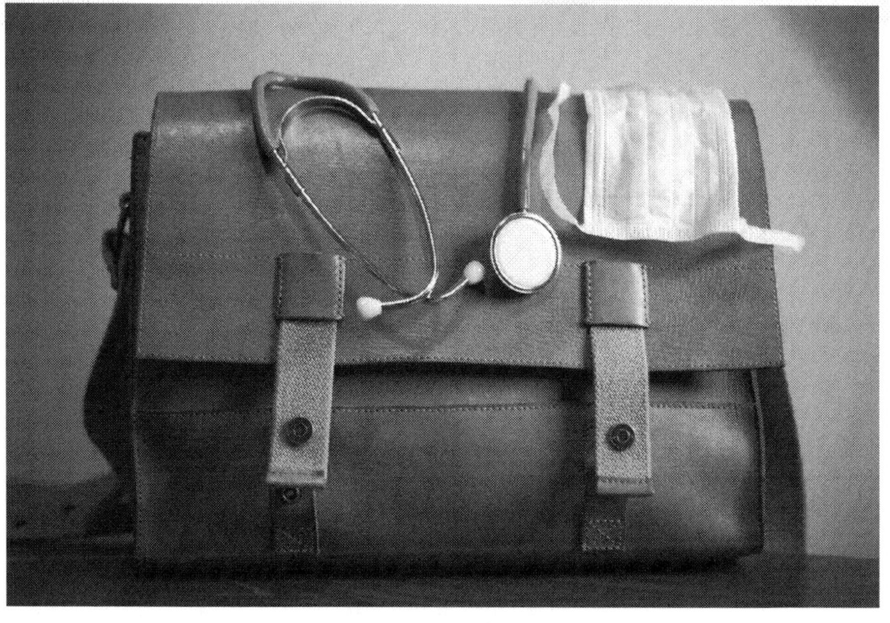

THE RIGHT EQUIPMENT

To succeed at a job, you need the right equipment. A lumberjack trying to cut down a tree with a steak knife wouldn't accomplish much; the same goes for the medic. Antibiotics may prevent or treat infection, but they won't stop bleeding. An effective medic has amassed a stockpile of medical supplies that can handle a variety of health issues.

How much do you need? Well, that depends. Are you expecting to be exposed to an epidemic disease? Are you traveling in hostile terrain or climate, or perhaps in areas where the inhabitants themselves are hostile? You may never have to deal with, for example, a major hemorrhage in remote but stable settings. In other situations, your people may be constantly at risk for major trauma.

When it comes to determining the amount of supplies needed, the answer is: The more the better. You don't know how long you might have to function without access to modern medical care. As such, you may search for kits that advertise the ability to handle groups of 50 or 100 people. If you look at the contents, however, you see immediately that the manufacturers are assuming that everyone is healthy and you're in a safe environment. In times of trouble, you'll expend "100 people's worth" of supplies in short order.

It's important to note that the value of many medical supplies depends largely on the knowledge and skill that the user has obtained through study and practice. A blood pressure cuff isn't very useful to someone who doesn't know how to take a blood pressure.

Concentrate first on obtaining items that you know how to use, and then purchase more advanced equipment as you learn more skills. Hopefully, you know more about antibiotics now than when you first opened this book.

Of course, there is the possibility that, at one point or another, a medical professional with training to use advanced supplies may join your group. Having a wider variety of materials in your kit will help that person become a valuable asset.

Over time, you'll be using the items you have to deal with injuries and illness. Some may be replaceable; others will not. It's wise to keep a running inventory of supplies on hand so you can replace them, if possible, as needed.

Don't forget that many items can be improvised; a bandanna can serve as a sling, an ironing board as a stretcher, or thin fishing line and a sewing needle as suturing equipment. A careful inspection of your own home would probably turn up lots of items that can be adapted to medical use. Look with a creative eye and you'll be surprised at how many medical issues you are already equipped to deal with.

The Medic Bag

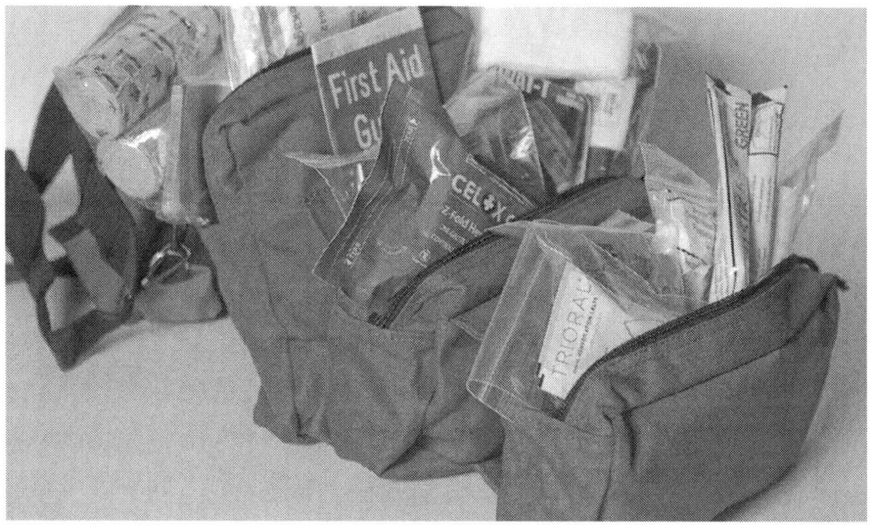

Trauma Medium Kit Bag

Once you have accumulated a significant number of medical supplies, you have to organize them for easy access in emergencies. If you're staying in place, an unused closet or pantry may suffice. In some settings, however, you're on the move and your supplies must be mobile as well.

Many sources will tell you what to put in a medical kit, but few discuss the medical bag that will contain all these supplies. Without a place to put your medical supplies, they will, most likely, be stored haphazardly in a way that prevents easy access to the items you may need in a hurry. This wastes precious time when someone's life may hang in the balance.

One important aspect of choosing a bag that fits your needs is size. You should assess your needs to determine which size bag is right for you. The factors that go into this decision include:

- Are you staying in place or on the move?
- How many people are you responsible for? How healthy are they?
- How long will you be the medical resource for your family or group?
- Are you in an area that is potentially dangerous?
- What climate should you be prepared for?
- What medical issues will you be most likely to encounter?
- Can you depend on nearby clean water?
- How many medical supplies do you have?

The additional question asked by this book is: Are you at risk for infection? Is there an epidemic raging in the area?

It's probable that some in your group must separate to perform varying tasks of daily survival in off-grid settings. Which basic medical supplies should every family member carry in case the medic isn't present at the time of injury? What are more advanced supplies that the medic should carry?

You might start by having members of your group carry an **IFAK** (Individual First Aid Kit) whenever they're away from your retreat or base camp. The family medic carries more advanced items in a larger bag.

The best medic bags are sturdy and water-resistant with lots of clear or mesh pockets. These bags have everything you'll need in plain sight if packed right, something you'll appreciate if an emergency requires rapid action. If someone's injured, you never want to ask yourself: "Where'd I put the tourniquet?," or "Where'd I put the burn dressings?"

Although mesh or clear plastic compartments are great, most bags come with at least some closed pouches. These could be used for non-emergency items, like certain medicines, water filters, etc. Consider putting items in groups based on the issues they handle.

The important thing is to have the medical kit make sense for you. This might mean taking an already packed kit like one of ours at store.doomand-bloom.net and moving things around so that the arrangement seems natural for your purposes. The items in our kits are placed in locations intuitive for us but that doesn't mean they shouldn't be adjusted to match your needs. Don't take your commercially-produced medical kit and put it in your closet; take it apart and make it your own.

By the way, medical bags don't necessarily have to be commercially-produced; a tool box or other item that sets up your supplies in an organized way is all that is needed. Just be aware that you may have to carry it to where an emergency is taking place.

MEDICAL KITS

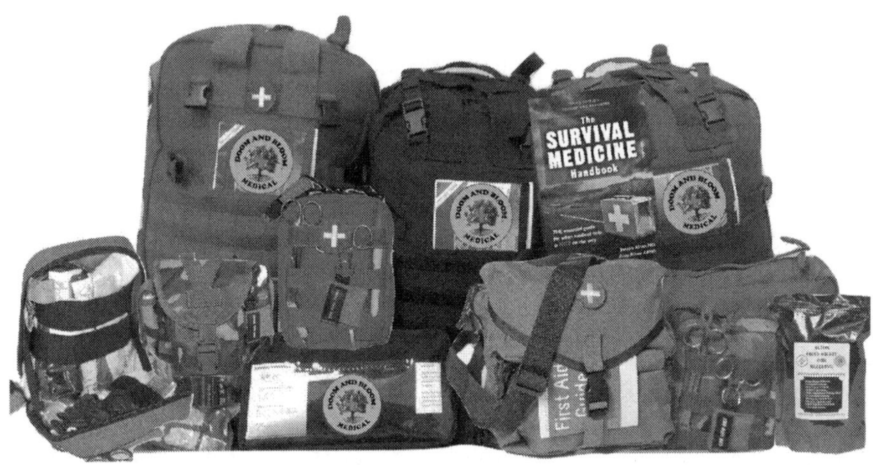

Grab N Go® Kits designed by the Altons

Once you have decided on a medic bag, it's time to equip it with the things you'll need to be medically prepared. You, hopefully, will already have some of these supplies.

Most people will search for an already-completed kit and, indeed, we even design such kits ourselves for our website. Many other commercial first aid kits are fine for a single mishap, but not enough to handle your long-term role as family medic in a disaster or other austere setting. Always have more medical supplies than you think you need. You may be responsible for more people than you expect.

There are three levels of medical kits that we will identify and for which we'll list our preferences for content:

- The individual first aid kit, also called an "IFAK"
- The "family kit"
- The "field hospital"

The lightest kit is the individual first aid kit or IFAK. Every member of a group carries this kit; it allows for treatment of some common issues encountered in the wilderness or when traveling. This kit is more effective when every member of a group is given some medical training, as you may not always be present when an injury occurs.

The IFAK is certainly useful to the person carrying it, but also the medic as a source of supply. If someone is injured, the medic may first use items from the injured party's kit. This serves as a resource multiplier and allows healthcare personnel to carry the more advanced equipment in their pack. One example of a useful IFAK item is a tourniquet.

The second kit listed below is the "family kit": This kit has a lot of supplies but should be mobile enough to fit in a large dedicated backpack. The items will suffice as a medical "bug-out" kit for a couple and their children. It is, in our opinion, the minimum amount of equipment that a head of household would need to handle common emergencies in a long-term survival situation.

A family kit is meant to be sufficient to fully handle injuries and illnesses for a small number of people. This set requires a designated individual (probably you) to transport it when changes of location are necessary. A typical item for this kit would be a moldable 36-inch splint.

The third kit is the "field hospital." It will contain everything that you have stockpiled for the long-term care of a family or group. This is too much material to be carried; it is meant to be kept at a retreat or other static location. As such, items here would include furniture like a number of cots, dedicated bedding, plastic sheeting, and work surfaces.

Don't feel intimidated by the sheer volume of supplies listed in the more advanced kits. Few of us have the resources or skills to purchase and effectively use every single item. If you can put together a good family kit, you will have accomplished a great deal. Evaluate the scenario to identify the subset of items that would be most useful.

Here are the supplies we recommend for each kit (description or brand names in parenthesis when appropriate). How many can you check off as already part of your supplies?

The IFAK (Individual First Aid Kit)

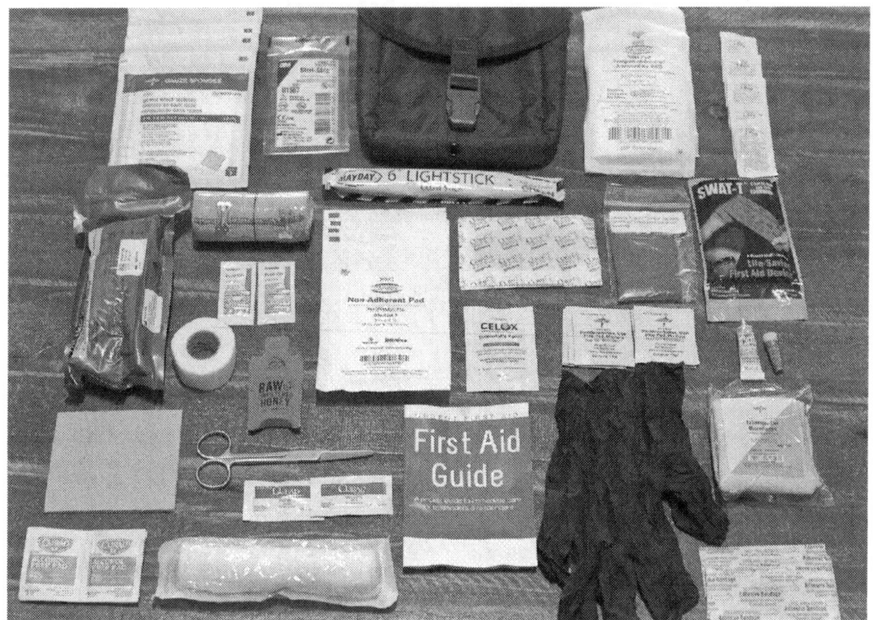

Ultimate Compact First Aid Trauma Kit Grab N Go®

- o Nitrile gloves (hypoallergenic)
- o Cold packs/Hot packs, instant and/or reusable
- o Scalpels and/or field knife
- o Elastic (Ace) Wraps
- o Pressure Dressings
- o Celox or Quikclot hemostatic clotting agents (stops moderate to severe bleeding in wounds)
- o Tourniquets (CAT, SOF-T, and SWAT)
- o Compressed vacuum-packed sterile Gauze

- Steri-Strips (to close small lacerations when appropriate)
- Tincture of Benzoin (glue-like substance to help strips stick to skin)
- Iris Scissors
- Hemostat Clamp 5," Straight or Curved
- 3-0 Nylon or Silk Suture
- Super Glue or medical glue
- Tweezers
- Penlight (to check pupils)
- Bandage scissors 7.25" Stainless steel (better) or EMT scissors
- Adhesive Bandages, various sizes (non-latex if possible)
- ABD pads, various sizes
- Gauze dressings sterile and non-sterile, various sizes
- Non-Stick sterile dressings (Telfa type), various sizes
- Gauze rolls sterile (Kerlix), various sizes
- Moleskin or other blister pads
- Mylar blankets
- Cloth or paper medical tape
- Duct tape
- Triangular bandage with safety pins, and bandannas
- Ammonia inhalants
- Antibiotic ointment or creams, (Bacitracin or Neomycin)
- Antiseptic wipes (Alcohol, Betadine, BZK)
- Burn gel and hydrocortisone cream
- Sting relief wipes
- Hand sanitizer
- Lip balm
- Sunscreen
- Ibuprofen
- Diphenhydramine (Benadryl)
- Oral rehydration packets
- Waterproof paper and pencil

The Family Kit

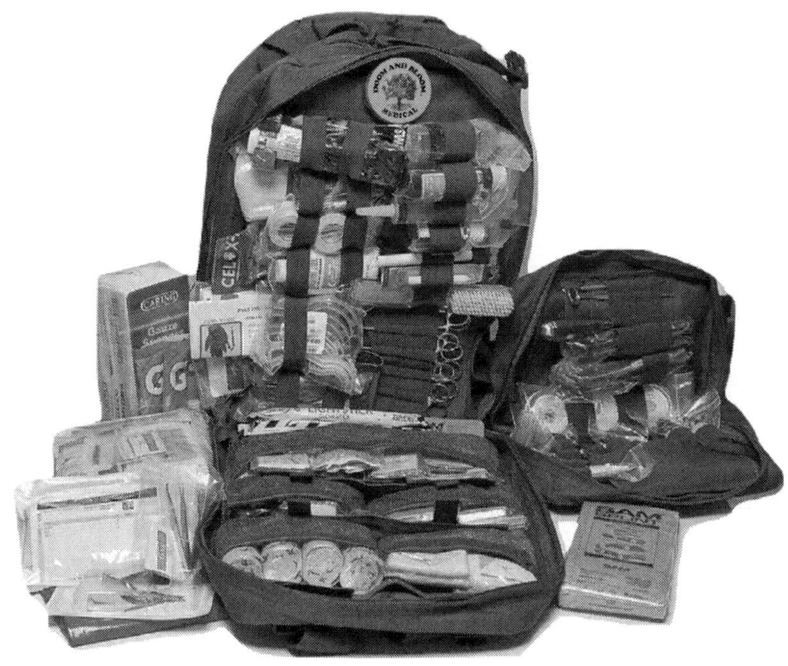

Ultimate Family Medical Survival Bag Grab N Go®

All of the above (some are mentioned again for emphasis) in greater quantity, plus:

- o First Aid Reference Book (Consider "The Survival Medicine Handbook: The Essential Guide for when Medical Help is Not on the Way")
- o Headlamps (for night or poor lighting conditions)
- o Instant Glucose and/or Raw Unprocessed Honey
- o Chest seals, vented (2 per injury to cover entry and exit wounds)
- o Oral airways (keeps airways open)
- o Nasal airways or "NPAs" (keeps airways open) and Surgical lube
- o Soap and/or Dr. Bronner's Castile liquid soap

- CPR shields
- Safety pins (large), Rubber Bands, and Paper Clips
- Scalpels and disposable blades
- Neck collars, various sizes
- Extra-large absorbent pads (ABD or other brand)
- Petrolatum/Xeroform dressings in various sizes
- Burn dressings (non-stick) and burn blankets
- Coban or other self-adhering wraps
- Liquid Bandage (Like New Skin)
- Medical tapes, various types (Elastoplast, silk, and paper) and sizes (1 inch, 2 inch etc.)
- Skin Tac liquid adhesive barrier (prepares skin for application of tapes, dressings and protects the skin with a hypo-allergenic sticky film) or equivalent skin prep wipes
- Moleskin or Spenco Second Skin Blister kit
- Styptic pencils (stops mild bleeding)
- Eye cups, eye pads or patches, and eye wash
- SAM splints, various sizes (can be shaped to fit the injured area)
- Triangular bandages (slings)
- Blood Pressure Cuff (sphygmomanometer)
- Stethoscope
- Bio Glo Strips (Fluorescein sodium Rx only)- used to stain the eye, and a Cobalt Blue light bulb to shine on the injured eye and allow visualization of cuts or foreign objects
- Cotton swabs (Q-tips), cotton balls, cotton-tipped applicators, cotton rounds
- Face masks (basic ear loop surgical and N95)
- Chest decompression needles
- Tongue depressors
- Magnifying glass
- Glow sticks

- Multi-tool (Swiss Army, etc.)
- Flashlights and extra batteries
- Paracord 550
- Ring cutter
- Kelly clamps, straight and curved in various sizes
- Needle holders
- Half circle sewing needles and silk thread
- Sutures in their many variations, such as:
- Vicryl; 0, 2-0, 4-0 (absorbable)
- Chromic 0, 2-0, 4-0 (absorbable)
- Silk, Nylon, and Prolene 0, 2-0, 3-0, 4-0 (non-absorbable)
- Disposal box for needles and other sharp waste
- Suture removal tray
- Surgical staplers and staple removers
- Iodoform sterile packing gauze
- Silver nitrate sticks and cautery pens
- Saline solution (can be homemade with recipe in this book)
- Irrigation syringes (60-100 ml is good) and irrigation cups (Zerowet)
- Hair combs (including special lice versions) and brushes
- Nail files, foot files and heel creams
- Thermometers (rectal, oral or ear)
- Hot water bottles and ice bags (both reusable)
- Ziploc bags, plastic wrap
- Aluminum foil (use to sharpen scissors, by cutting the foil several times)
- Cotton sheets (100% in white)
- Eye droppers and bulb syringes
- Measuring spoons and cups
- Antiseptic solutions in large and medium quantities (Betadine, Hibiclens, etc.)

- Hydrogen peroxide 3% and 6-7%
- Rubbing alcohol
- Nutritional supplements (Boost, Pediasure) vitamins, multi, and pregnancy vitamins
- Sunblock
- Lip balms
- Insect repellants
- Bactine or equivalent (for cuts and bug bites)
- Fels-Naptha or Zanfel soap (poison ivy, oak and sumac)
- Poison ivy wipes
- Hydrocortisone cream 1%
- Lidocaine cream or jelly 2.5% (topical anesthetic)
- Dermoplast spray or Solarcaine
- Medi-First burn spray (analgesic, antiseptic and liquid bandaid all in one)
- Biofreeze gel or cold freeze spray for intact skin only
- Acetaminophen/ibuprofen/aspirin
- Benadryl (diphenhydramine)
- Epinephrine (Epi-Pen, prescription injection for severe allergic reactions)
- Claritin (loratadine)
- Anti-nausea medication (meclizine hydrochloride 2.5mg tablets)
- Zofran or Dramamine (for nausea and vomiting)
- Ear and eye drops
- Cough syrup and lozenges/drops expectorants (to loosen up thick mucus)
- Decongestants (to move mucus out of the respiratory system)
- Vicks Vapo-Rub (or equivalent)
- Nebulizer, saline, tubing, mask or mouth piece (plus albuterol single dose liquid)

- o Sleep aids (like Alteril, Tylenol pm, melatonin, chamomile or valerian tea etc.)
- o Fiber supplements
- o Stool softeners and laxatives suppositories and finger cots
- o Beano, Gas-X or equivalent (to reduce gas formation with certain foods)
- o Imodium anti-diarrheal (loperamide)
- o Pepto-Bismol (bismuth subsalicylate)
- o Heartburn medications and natural treatments
- o Lice shampoo, lotion or creme rinse
- o Lice comb
- o Oral rehydration packets (or make yourself from recipe in this book)
- o Water purification tablets
- o Emergency water bag
- o Water filters, portable and large family size
- o Waterproof matches, lighters and other methods to start fires
- o Gold Bond foot powder
- o Calamine lotion
- o Burn cream (Silvadene), burn gel or other burn treatments with anesthetic
- o Colloidal silver (for external treatments) anti-fungal cream (terconazole)
- o Anti-fungal powder (Tinactin)
- o Fluconazole 100 or 150mg tablets (antifungal agent mentioned in this book)
- o Urinary pain reliever (Uristat or Azo tablets)
- o Wart removal cream/ointment/solution/freeze
- o Hemorrhoid cream or ointment (Preparation H)
- o Zinc oxide cream or ointment
- o A & d ointment
- o Vaseline petroleum jelly (use with gauze to make burn dressings)
- o Muscle rub (like Icy Hot or arnica salve)

- Tens unit or equivalent (muscle stimulation pain reliever machine)
- Oral antibiotics (discussed in this book)
- Radiation pills (Thyrosafe or equivalent, one box per person)
- PMS medication, like Pamprin (which acts as a mild diuretic also), and natural remedies
- Caffeine pills
- Natural equivalents of any the above; see natural medicine chapters
- Birth control accessories (condoms, birth control pills, cervical caps, etc.)
- Emergency obstetric kit (comes as a pack) and nitrazine strips (pH strips)
- Midwifery reference books
- Fetal electronic monitor or fetoscope
- Maxi pads and tampons (feminine hygiene; tampons for nose bleeds)
- Measuring tapes
- Paper, pencils, pens and permanent markers

Dental Tray:

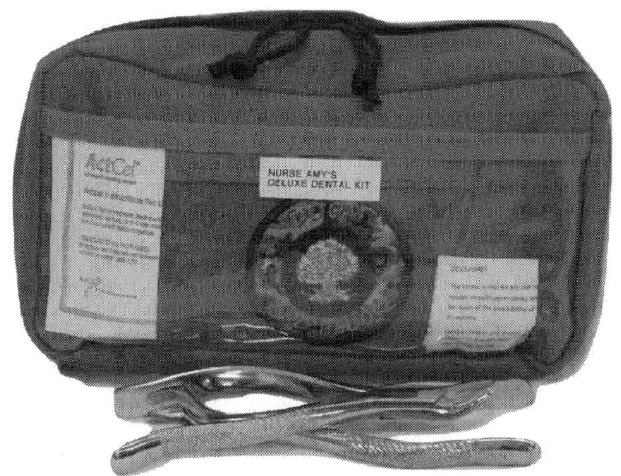

Deluxe Dental Kit Grab N Go®

- Cotton pellets and rolls dental mirror
- Tongue blades
- Toothpaste and toothbrushes
- Baking soda and peppermint oil
- Hydrogen peroxide 3% (oral rinse to treat or prevent gum issues)
- Syringes 12cc curved tip
- Dental scraper
- Dental pick and toothpicks
- Dental floss and dental wax
- Oral analgesics
- Canker sore tx (like Orajel or Hurricane gel)
- Clove bud oil (anesthetic for toothache)
- Zinc oxide (make a paste with oil of cloves and you get temporary dental cement), or...
- Commercial dental kits (Den-Temp, Cavit)
- Hank's solution (used to preserve viability in knocked-out teeth)
- Pill cups
- Scalpels, disposable
- 4-0 chromic sutures (absorbable) needle holder
- Gauze 2 x 2 inches
- Actcel hemostatic agent (stops dental bleeding, and dissolves naturally)
- Extraction equipment (several different extractors and elevators)
- Spoon excavator
- Generic or brand name ibuprofen
- Gloves, masks, and eye protection

Natural Remedy Supplies

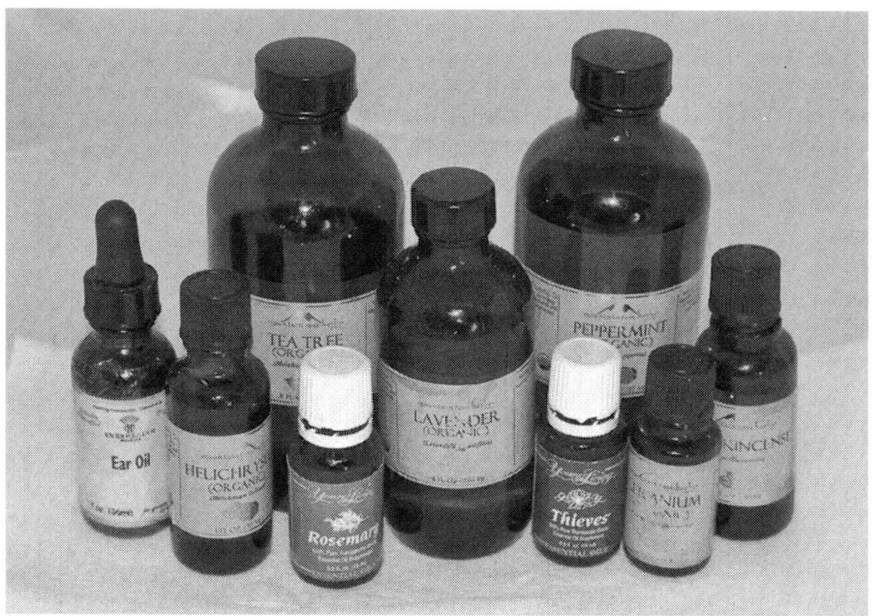

- Witch hazel and extract bag balm ointment drawing salve
- Raw unprocessed honey (local is best)
- Cayenne pepper powder (see medicinal garden chapter) aloe vera
- Herbal teas, tinctures
- Salves
- Essential oils
- Neti pot (use only with sterile solutions)
- Diffusers
- Medicinal herb and plant seeds (in long-term storage packaging)
- Herbal medicine reference books
- Gardening reference books
- Mortar and pestle
- Graters, stainless steel
- Clear and brown glass jars with lids

- Glass bottles (various sizes) green, brown and clear, with cork tops
- Metal tins, ½ ounce to 4 ounce sizes sealing wax
- Funnels, kitchen mesh strainers and cotton muslin bags
- Clocks and kitchen timers
- Kitchen scale
- Grain alcohol and vodkas (for making tinctures), other spirits as needed
- Copper distiller (to distill essential oils, etc.)
- Cheesecloth
- Coffee filters
- Tea ball infuser
- Coconut, olive, neem, sesame, shea nut oils
- Wheat germ, castor oils
- Grapeseed, soybean oils
- Vegetable glycerin, vitamin e oil, steric acid oils
- Grapefruit seed extract
- Citric acid
- White cosmetic clay (kaolin), makes an excellent poultice base
- Beeswax and pastilles
- Cocoa butter wax and wafers
- Shea butter
- Gelatin or vegetable capsules,
- Capsule making machine
- Teapots, coffee pots
- Coal tar shampoo
- Selenium shampoo
- Baking soda and corn starch
- Apple cider vinegar and white vinegar
- Epsom salts
- Sugar
- Salt

- Salt substitutes (part of rehydration formula)
- Cayenne pepper powder (for sore throat gargle and to help stop mild-mod bleeding)
- Saline nasal spray (or sterile homemade solution)

The Field Hospital

All of the above in larger quantities, plus:

- Extensive medical library
- Face shields
- Tyvek coveralls
- Hoodies
- Aprons
- Boots
- Long gloves
- Waterproof boots
- Goggles, indirect vented
- Treatment table, work counters
- Stretchers
- Cots or beds and chairs
- Bedside table
- Rolling stands
- Portable lights
- Waste bins
- Biohazard bags
- Trash bags
- Heavy plastic sheeting
- Duct tape
- Mosquito netting
- Portable large capacity tent or shelter
- White 100% cotton sheets and pillow cases

- Pillows with waterproof cases
- Blankets, towels, patient gowns basins, bowls and washcloths
- Portable shower or curtain for privacy and portable sinks
- Shampoo and conditioner
- Hair clips and rubber bands
- Nail brushes, emery boards and nail clippers
- Large capacity water filtration systems water pitcher and cups
- Lemon glycerin swabs or equivalent
- Disposable razors, or lots of blades
- Chux or other waterproof pads
- Bedpans and portable male urinals
- Laundry soap, bleach, buckets, mop handle, dedicated laundry scrub brushes
- Clothesline
- Scrub suits
- Fire extinguishers
- Extra reading glasses in various strengths
- Charting materials and forms
- Clip boards, pencils and pens (don't forget the sharpeners)
- Watch with a second hand and stopwatch
- Scales, newborn and adult sizes
- Resuscitation facemask with one-way valve
- Bag valve mask (Ambu-Bag)
- Endotracheal tube/ laryngoscope (allows you to breathe for patient)
- Portable defibrillator (expensive item also known as an "AED")
- Pulse oximeter (identifies oxygen status and pulse of patient; battery-powered)
- Oxygen concentrator, tubing, and face mask or nasal cannulas, with portable power source
- Portable EKG monitor (battery operated is preferred)
- Blood pressure monitors (battery operated, wrist sizes are handy)

- Otoscope and ophthalmoscope—(instruments to look into ears and eyes)
- Microscope
- Glucose monitor
- Urine test strips and Hemoccult test strips
- Pregnancy test kits
- Sterile drapes
- Portable refrigerator A/C and D/C capacity
- Air splints (arm/long-leg/short-leg)
- Plaster of Paris cast kits (to make casts for fractures) adult and pediatric
- Cast removal tools
- Crutches, walking canes, wheelchair
- Drain and IV sponges (dressings with a slit cutout)
- Tegaderm film dressing
- IV equipment, such as:
- Normal Saline (has the longest shelf life)
- Ringer's lactate IV solutions
- IV tubing sets—maxi-sets + standard sets
- Blood collection bags + filter transfusion sets
- Syringes 2/5/10/20 ml
- Needles 20/22/24 gauge
- IV start kits with Tegaderm dressings
- Angiocath IV needles: 16/18/20/24 gauge
- Paper tape (1/2 or 1 inch) to secure IV lines
- IV stands (to hang fluid bottles)
- Enema bags
- Paracord (various uses)
- Assorted hemostats and other clamps (curved and straight)
- Scalpel handle with blades (sizes 10, 11, 15) and/or disposable
- Triage tags (for mass casualty incidents)

- o Autoclave or pressure cooker (to sterilize instruments and other items)
- o Stainless steel tongs (to place inside sterilizer and use to pick out sterilized instruments)
- o Self-sealing sterilization pouches with indicator strips
- o Ultraviolet sterilization wand or unit
- o Vacuum bags and food saver
- o Cidex solution or equivalent (for cleaning instruments)
- o Dedicated scrub brushes for cleaning instruments only
- o Surgical trays and bowls, stainless steel only
- o Heavy trash bags and biohazard bags, various sizes
- o Human remains pouch with ID cards or tags
- o Shovels and hatchets
- o Bucket, scrub brushes and mop (to clean hospital surfaces and floors)
- o Bleach and/or pool shock (to DIY bleach)
- o Quick lime powder (sanitation of human waste)
- o Toilet paper, tissues and paper towels
- o Pill bottles and labels
- o Books, deck of cards, games, music, paper, pens, colored pencils/crayons and activity books (for patients to pass the time)
- o Poster board, permanent markers and red duct tape, for signage outside the "hospital"

Surgery Tray Items:

- o Sterile gloves
- o Sterile towels
- o Scrub brushes in sterile single packages
- o Hibiclens antiseptic surgical scrub (to clean skin before invasive procedures)
- o Mayo scissors

- Metzenbaum scissors
- Needle holders, sterile in various sizes
- Surgical marking pens
- Suction pump with internal 12v rechargeable battery
- Nasogastric tubes (to pump a stomach)
- Nasal speculum (to look up the nose)
- 1% or 2% Lidocaine (prescription local anesthetic in injectable form)
- Sterile irrigation syringes (for flushing wounds during procedures)
- Sterile lap sponges and large quantity of dressings and gauze
- Obstetric forceps (for difficult deliveries)
- Vaginal **speculums**, small to ex-large sizes
- Uterine **curettes** (for miscarriages or retained placentas after childbirth, various sizes)
- Uterine "sound" (checks depth of uterine canal)
- Uterine dilators (allows removal of retained products of conception in miscarriages)
- Chromic **catgut** suture and surgical tray (vaginal laceration repair)
- Bone saw kit (for amputations)
- Chest tube set-up (must have some way that connects to bedside suction)
- Penrose and Jackson-Pratt drains (to allow blood and pus to drain from wounds)

Antibiotics

A selection of various antibiotics as described in this book:

- Amoxicillin 250 mg
- Amoxicillin 500 mg
- Ampicillin 250 mg
- Cephalexin 250 mg
- Cephalexin 500 mg

- Metronidazole 250 mg
- Metronidazole 500 mg
- Penicillin 250 mg
- Penicillin 500 mg
- Ciprofloxacin 250 mg
- Ciprofloxacin 500 mg
- Clindamycin 150 mg
- Minocycline 50 Or 100 mg
- Erythromycin 250 mg
- Doxycycline 100 mg
- Doxycycline 100 mg
- Sulfamethoxazole 400 mg/Trimethoprim 80mg
- Sulfamethoxazole 800 mg/Trimethoprim 160mg
- Azithromycin 250 mg
- Fluconazole 100 mg

Additional Prescription Medications

- Medrol Dose packs (oral steroids)
- Epi Pens and Inhalers (Ventolin)
- Metformin 500 mg, 1000 mg tablets
- Salbutamol Inhalers (for asthma/severe allergic reactions)
- Antibiotic and Anesthetic, Eye ointment/drops and Ear drops
- Oral Contraceptive Pills
- Ceftriaxone, IV antibiotic
- Diazepam IV (Valium) sedative to treat seizures
- Diazepam in oral form, sedative
- Alprazolam, oral anti-anxiety agent
- Oxytocin (Pitocin) IV for post-delivery hemorrhage
- Percocet, (oxycodone with paracetamol/acetaminophen), strong oral pain medicine
- Morphine Sulfate or Demerol (strong injectable pain medicine)

- o Tramadol (stronger pain medicine)

If you have any children in your family, make sure you have pediatric versions of both supplies and medications. Also, if anyone in your family or group has specific medications they are currently taking, make every effort to have a supply on hand.

There are so many medical items on the market that we're sure there is something we might have missed. The important thing is to accumulate supplies and equipment that you will feel competent using in the event of an illness or an injury.

Some of the above supplies, such as stretchers and tourniquets, can be improvised using common household items. For example, duct tape can be used as a butterfly dressing to close wounds and Paracord can be used to make a rope stretcher.

It should be noted that many of the advanced items are probably useful only in the hands of an experienced surgeon, and could be very dangerous otherwise. Why should you have medical or dental items that are beyond your pay grade? Because you never know when a medical professional experienced in their use might stumble across your threshold.

Of course, some of the supplies listed would be more successful in their purpose with an intact power grid. These items represent a wish list of what we would want if we were taking care of an entire community.

You should not feel that the more advanced supply lists are your responsibility to accumulate alone. Your entire family or group should contribute to stockpiling supplies under the medic's coordination. The same goes for all the medical skills that I've listed. To learn everything would take more than even a formally-trained physician can accomplish in a lifetime of study. Concentrate on the items that you are most likely to use regularly and be grateful for the assistance from others with education and skills.

AN OPEN LETTER TO HEALTHCARE PROVIDERS ABOUT DISASTER PREPAREDNESS

This is a letter that any person concerned about disasters can present to their physician. It discusses what happens to the unprepared in situations and asks for cooperation in helping patients obtain needed medicines. Feel free to print it and present it to your family physician if you think it would help them to better understand preparedness issues.

To my fellow physicians:

I am a Fellow of both the American College of Surgeons and the American College of OB/GYN, recently retired, and I am writing this letter in an effort to inform you about the importance of improving the level of medical preparedness in your patient population.

We live in uncertain times, and more and more people are becoming concerned about what would happen in the event of a major disaster. From natural events to national emergencies, there are circumstances where medical personnel may be overwhelmed by the number of victims requiring medical aid. In these situations, many of your patients will be unable to reach you and may find themselves as the sole medical resource available to sick or injured members of their families.

In the aftermath of Hurricane Katrina in 2005, disaster medical assistance teams were overwhelmed by the number of victims requiring medical help. In such a scenario, it stands to reason that your patients would benefit from your help in preparing them to deal with the problems they would face.

In this era of high technology, we may have expectations that our resources will always be sufficient to meet our emergency needs. Recent history has proven otherwise, and it may be time for us, as physicians, to take an active stand to prepare our patients for disasters; in this way, they can function as assets to their family if you or emergency medical personnel are not available.

Few medical offices provide information regarding the types and quantities of medical supplies that are recommended for the average household. These are my suggestions: Consider your area's likely needs for the disasters that might befall it, and print lists of items that you would advise your patients to have in their homes.

Provide resources for your patient so that they will have the data necessary to deal with health issues likely in natural disasters, epidemics, and other events. You might consider directing them to sites recommended by the federal government for emergency preparedness, such as www.ready.gov; there, they will find advice that may help increase their chances of surviving natural calamities and other disasters.

For your individual patients, especially those with chronic medical problems, you might consider providing the opportunity for them to keep a supply of needed medications by offering them an extra prescription to fill. In this manner, you can assure that your patients will have enough medicine to get them through situations which prevent them from contacting you in times of trouble.

I'm not asking you to abandon your responsibility to them by throwing prescriptions at them; I am simply suggesting that they would benefit from having some extra supplies available to deal with unforeseen circumstances. Also, consider listing recommended over-the-counter medications that would be useful to have on hand.

Our purpose as physicians is to improve the health of our people while doing no harm. Many doctors dedicate their entire lives to this purpose, and we must work to preserve the well-being of our patients in bad times as well as good times.

The worst nightmare of your patients is the inability to reach you in a major disaster; help them become better prepared to deal with medical emergencies with education, compassion, and understanding.

Thank you for all you do to keep your patients healthy, and for your time and attention in reading this letter.

—Joseph Alton, M.D., F.A.C.S., F.A.C.O.G.

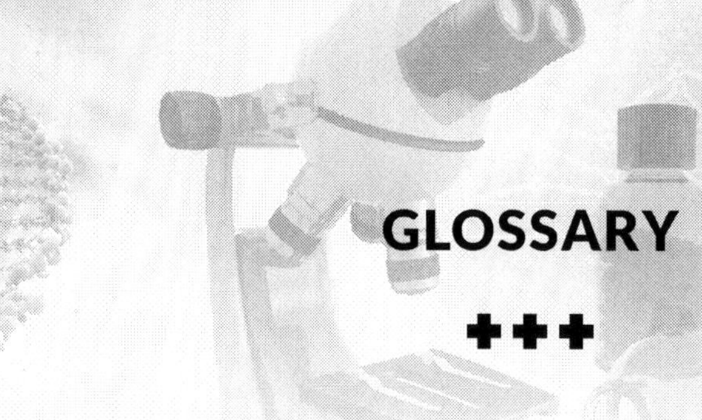

GLOSSARY

✚✚✚

ABSCESS: A collection of pus.

AEROBIC: Organisms that require the presence of oxygen to survive.

ALLERGEN: A substance that induces an allergy.

ALLERGY: An exaggerated immune response by the body to a substance to which it has become hypersensitive.

ALVEOLI: Small air sacs in lung tissue that absorb oxygen from the air.

AMEBIASIS: A form of dysentery caused by Entamoeba histolytica.

ANAEROBIC: Organisms that don't require the presence of oxygen to survive.

ANAPHYLACTIC SHOCK: A severe allergy which may affect the entire body and become life-threatening.

ANEMIA: Blood condition characterized by a low amount of red blood cells.

ANTHRAX: Bacteria found in soil that often infects livestock, but also used as a biological weapon against humans.

ANTIBIOTICS: A medicine that inhibits the growth of or destroys certain pathogens.

ANTIBODIES: A Y-shaped protein produced in the blood as a response to a specific antigen which the body recognizes as alien.

ANTIGENS: A toxin or other foreign substance which induces the production of antibodies and other immune responses.

ANTIMYCOTIC: A drug that inhibits or kills fungi.

ANTISEPTIC: A substance that inhibits the growth or action of microbes in or on living tissue.

ANTITOXIN: An antibody produced in response to the presence of a toxin.

APNEA: A cessation, usually temporary, in breathing.

APPENDICITIS: Inflammation of the appendix.

ASCARIS: A type of parasitic intestinal worm.

ASYMPTOMATIC: Having no clear signs or symptoms of a disease or infection.

AUSTERE: Lacking in modern facilities, equipment, or comforts.

AVULSION: A tearing away of tissue due to trauma.

BACILLI: Bacteria that are cylindrical in shape. These may exist singly, in pairs, in chains, or other combinations.

BACTERIA: Single-celled prokaryotic microorganisms which have cell walls but lack organelles and an organized nucleus.

BACTERIAL RESISTANCE: The development of traits in a bacterial species that make it less likely to be eliminated by an antibiotic.

BACTERICIDAL: Having the ability to kill bacteria outright.

BACTERIOSTATIC: Inhibiting bacterial growth and/or reproduction.

BACTERIUM: Singular form of "bacteria."

BETA-LACTAM RING: A chemical structure that is part of the molecule of drugs in the penicillin and cephalosporin family.

BINARY FISSION: A form of reproduction in bacteria and other prokaryotes that involves the splitting of a parent cell into two independent cells.

BLACK DEATH: Commonly used name for outbreaks of Yersinia Pestis, or "Plague."

BOTULISM: Infection caused by toxins produced by the bacterium Clostridium botulinum.

BRADYCARDIA: A slow heart rate (less than 60).

BROAD SPECTRUM: Effective against a large variety of organisms.

BRONCHITIS: An inflammation of the airways leading from the windpipe (trachea) to the lungs.

BRUDZINSKI'S SIGN: Finding on exam suggestive of meningitis: When flexing the neck, the hip and legs flex as well.

BUBOES: Lumps seen in the groins and armpits of victims of the bubonic plague.

BUBONIC PLAGUE: The most common form of plague.

BULLAE: fluid-1filled skin lesions similar to blisters. .

CAMPYLOBACTER: Common bacterial cause of food poisoning.

CAPSID: The protein coat of a virus.

CARRIER: One who harbors a pathogen on their body without symptoms.

CATGUT: Suture material actually made from the intestinal lining of sheep and cattle.

CDC: Short term for the Centers for Disease Control and Prevention.

CELL-MEDIATED IMMUNITY: The immune response that identifies and destroys infected cells.

CELLULITE: Skin dimpling of soft tissue on the buttocks, legs, and elsewhere not associated with infection.

CELLULITIS: Infection of soft tissue.

CHALAZION: A blocked gland under the eyelid unrelated to infection.

CHANCRE: The skin ulcer seen in primary syphilis.

CHITIN: A fibrous carbohydrate that is found in fungal cell walls as well as the exoskeletons of spiders, insects, and crustaceans.

CHLAMYDIA: Sexually transmitted disease caused by the bacteria Chlamydia trachomatis.

CHLOROPLAST: An organelle in plants which conducts photosynthesis.

CHOLERA: An infectious disease in areas of poor sanitation characterized by severe diarrhea.

CHROMOSOME: A threadlike structure carrying genetic information in the form of genes.

CLINICAL INFECTION: An infection that shows physical signs and symptoms.

COCCI: Bacteria that are round or oval-shaped. These may exist singly, in pairs, in chains, or other combinations.

COHORTING: placement of patients infected with the same pathogens in the same designated unit or ward.

COLONIZATION: the presence of pathogenic bacteria on a body surface (like on the skin, mouth, intestines or airway) without causing clinical evidence of infection.

COMMENSALISTIC: A relationship between two species where one benefits with aiding or harming the other.

CONGENITAL: Existing at birth.

CONJUNCTIVITIS: Inflammation of the membrane that covers the white of the eye, also called "Pink Eye."

CONSUMPTION: Term given to Tuberculosis due to victims having the appearance of being "consumed" by the disease.

CONTAGION: The communication of disease from one person to another.

CONTRAINDICATION: A factor which would eliminate a drug as a candidate to treat an infection or condition.

CROSS-REACTIVE: A similarity in action or other characteristic between two different species of antibiotic.

CROUP: Respiratory illness in children, usually caused by a virus.

CRYPTOSPORIDIOSIS: Infection caused by drinking contaminated water containing the protozoan Cryptosporidium.

CULTURES: A method of multiplying microbial organisms by letting them reproduce under controlled laboratory conditions.

CURETTE: a surgical instrument used to remove material by a scraping action.

CUTANEOUS: Relating to the skin.

CYANOBACTERIA: Prokaryotic microorganisms related to bacteria but capable of photosynthesis. The earliest known life forms on Earth.

CYST: A hollow structure in an organ that is filled with fluid. Alternatively, a tough protective capsule enclosing the larva of a parasitic worm or the resting stage of certain microbes.

CYSTITIS: Infection of the bladder.

DAKIN'S SOLUTION: Time-honored mixture of water, bleach, and baking soda still used to prevent infection in open wounds.

DEBRIDEMENT: The act of surgically removing dead tissue from a wound.

DEFINITIVE THERAPY: The treatment deemed to be most affective against a specific organism for a specific ailment, usually identified with the help of lab tests and other technology.

DERMIS: The deep layer of the skin.

DIAGNOSIS: Determination of the nature or cause of a disease.

DIPHTHERIA: Highly contagious infection characterized by inflammation of the mucous membranes.

DISINFECTANT: A substances that destroy microbes on counters and other inanimate objects.

DRUG OF CHOICE: The medication currently recommended by conventional medicine to treat a certain condition.

DYSENTERY: Epidemic infection caused by bacteria in the Shigella species.

DYSURIA: Painful urination.

E. COLI: Bacterial species that exists in benign and virulent strains.

ELECTRON MICROSCOPE: An instrument that allows visualization of objects smaller than what can be seen by light microscopes.

EMPIRICAL THERAPY: Use of antibiotics to treat an infection before the specific causative organism has been identified with laboratory tests.

ENDEMIC: Disease constantly present in a particular region.

EPIDEMIC: Disease that suddenly appears in outbreaks in a particular region.

EPIDERMIS: The superficial layer of the skin.

ERYTHEMA: Redness in an area

ERYTHEMA MIGRANS: A rash that spreads with time commonly seen with Lyme disease.

EUKARYOTE: An organism consisting of a cell or cells in which the genetic material is DNA in the form of chromosomes contained within a nucleus. Include all life forms other than bacteria and cyanobacteria.

EXPIRATION DATE: The last date in which a pharmaceutical manufacturer will guarantee 100% of a medication.

EXUDATE: A mass of cells and fluid that seeps out of areas of inflammation.

FILAMENTOUS BACTERIA: Bacteria with branching threadlike structures called hyphae.

FISTULAS: Tunnels in the skin that connect affected organs to each other or to the skin surface.

FLAGELLUM: A simple threadlike structure that enables locomotion for many protozoa and bacteria.

FONTANELLE: The "soft spot" on the top of the heads of infants due to unfused skull bones.

FOOD POISONING: Any of a number of illnesses caused by exposure to poor prepared food.

FREQUENCY: Having to urinate frequently.

FUNGI: Eukaryotic organisms that includes microorganisms such as yeasts and molds.

FUNGUS: Singular form of "Fungi."

GERM: A microorganism, especially one which causes disease.

GERM THEORY OF DISEASE: The hypothesis that some diseases are caused by microbes.

GINGIVITIS: An inflammation of the gums.

GONORRHEA: Sexually transmitted disease caused by the bacteria *Neisseria gonorrheae.*

GRAM STAIN: A technique for a simple classification of bacteria formulated by the Danish Scientist Hans Gram.

GRAM-NEGATIVE: Bacteria that lose the crystal violet stain (and take the color of the red counterstain) in Gram's method of staining; bacteria that have a cell wall composed of a thin layer of peptidoglycan.

GRAM-POSITIVE: Bacteria that retain the purple color of the crystal violet stain in the Gram stain; bacteria that have a cell wall composed of a thick layer of peptidoglycan.

GRANULATION: The natural healing process of an open wound over time.

HELMINTHS: Parasitic worms that may cause harmful effects on their hosts.

HEMOPTYSIS: The coughing up of blood.

HERBALISM: The study or practice of the medicinal and therapeutic use of plants.

HERD IMMUNITY: The protection conferred to a non-immune individual by being in the midst of a population which is immune to a particular disease or infection.

HESITANCY: Difficulty with starting the stream of urine.

HIDRADENITIS SUPPURATIVA: Infection of soft tissues characterized by blocked sweat glands, frequently becoming infected with bacteria.

HOOKWORM: An intestinal worm that can also enter a human host through a break in the skin.

HUMORAL IMMUNITY: The immune response that eliminates antigens found in blood.

HYPHAE: Each of the branching filaments that make up the mycelium of a fungus.

IMMUNE-COMPROMISED: Lacking in immune defense against infectious disease.

IMMUNITY: The ability of an organism to resist a particular infection or toxin.

IMPETIGO: Skin infection characterized by red sores that burst, ooze yellow exudate, and then crust over.

INCISION AND DRAINAGE: Procedure in which a scalpel is use to incise the skin and drain an abscess.

INCLUSION CYSTS: A structure formed by the inclusion of lining in areas like the oral or nasal cavity.

INCUBATION PERIOD: The amount of time between exposure to a bacteria and physical signs and symptoms.

INDICATION: The infection or condition for which a drug is used.

INFECTION: The invasion of a living being by an organism which can cause disease.

INFESTATION: The presence of a large number of organisms, usually insects or animals, that cause disease or render the host unhealthy.

INTERACTIONS: The way that a drug's effect is changed by combining it with another drug (or other substance).

IRRIGATION: Washing a wound with a forceful stream of water or other fluid.

JAUNDICE: Yellowing of the skin and eyes caused by liver dysfunction.

KERNIG'S SIGN: Discomfort experienced by meningitis victims when extending the knee from a flexed position.

LARYNGOTRACHEOBRONCHITIS: Respiratory infection, commonly caused by a virus, seen in children.

LATENT: Present in the body and capable of emerging as a full-fledged illness.

LEUKOCYTES: White blood cells involved in protecting against infection.

LIGHT MICROSCOPE: An instrument that uses focused light and lenses to magnify a specimen, usually a cell.

LOADING DOSE: A stronger dose given at the very beginning of treatment to more rapidly achieve a therapeutic level of medicine in the body.

LOCALIZED INFECTION: An infection that stays in one area or body organ.

LOCKJAW: A manifestation of tetanus that is characterized by rigid spasms of the jaw muscles.

LONG-TERM IMMUNITY: The protection conferred by the "memory" that a body has of an offending organism; for example, the protection conferred by a vaccination against a certain disease.

LYME DISEASE: infectious disease spread by the bites of ticks.

MACROSCOPIC: Large enough to see with the naked eye.

MALAISE: A general feeling of ill health often seen with infections.

MALARIA: Infectious disease, often endemic, caused by protozoans and transmitted by mosquitoes.

MASTITIS: An infection of breast tissue commonly seen in nursing mothers.

MCBURNEY'S POINT: An area in the right lower quadrant of the abdomen where pain suggests an inflammation of the appendix.

MEDIC: The individual in a group who takes responsibility for the health of others.

MENINGES: Protective covering of the brain and spinal cord.

MENINGITIS: An infection of the protective covering of the brain and spinal cord.

METABOLISM: The processes that occur within a living organism in order to maintain life.

MICROBE: An organism too small to be seen with the naked eye.

MICROORGANISM: An organism too small to be seen with the naked eye.

MICROSCOPIC: Too small to be seen with the naked eye.

MITOSIS: Eukaryote cell reproduction by splitting into two "daughter" cells.

MORTALITY RATE: the number of deaths compared to the total number of cases

MRSA: A strain of Staphylococcus aureus that is resistant to Methicillin and certain other antibiotics.

MUCOUS MEMBRANE: Tissue which lines many body cavities and tubular organs including the GI and respiratory tracts.

MYCELIA: A network of fine filaments that make up (usually) a fungus, but also certain bacteria.

MYCELIUM: Singular form of mycelia.

MYCOPLASMA PNEUMONIAE: Type of bacterial respiratory infection commonly known as "walking pneumonia," as it is often not severe enough in nature to cause a patient to be bedridden.

MYCOSES: Fungal infections.

NARROW SPECTRUM: Effective against only a limited range of organisms.

NATURAL IMMUNITY: The resistance of an individual or an entire species against an infection or disease. Lack of natural immunity caused large numbers of Native Americans to succumb to smallpox when Europeans arrived in the New World.

NECROSIS: Tissue death due to disease, injury, loss of blood supply.

NECROTIZING FASCIITIS: An extreme form of cellulitis that destroys tissues.

NON-PHARMACEUTICAL INTERVENTION: A strategy to prevent infection that does not involve drugs.

NORMAL FLORA: Organisms that are normally present in or on the body without causing ill effect.

NUCLEUS: An organelle containing the genetic material in eukaryotic organisms.

ORGANELLES: Any of a number of organized or specialized structures within a living cell.

OTITIS: An infection of the ear canal which may be external (otitis externa), in the middle ear (otitis media) or internal (otitis interna).

OTOSCOPE: An instrument used to examine the ear canal.

PANDEMIC: Epidemic disease that after a number of geographic areas.

PARASITIC: A relationship between two species where one benefits at the expense of another.

PAROXYSMS: Coughing fits seen in whooping cough and other respiratory infections.

PATHOGEN: An organism which can cause disease.

PEPTIDOGLYCAN: A substance forming the cell walls of many bacteria.

PERITONITIS: Inflammation of the lining of the abdominal cavity.

PERTUSSIS: Highly contagious disease characterized by coughing fits.

PETECHIAE: Small red or purple spots caused by bleeding into the skin, eye, or other organ.

PHARYNGITIS: Inflammation of the throat.

PHOTOSYNTHESIS: The process by which green plants and some other organisms use sunlight to synthesize foods from carbon dioxide and water, generating oxygen as a by-product.

PILI: Hair-like structures on a bacterium that, among other things, help it attach to other cells.

PILONIDAL CYSTS: A hollow structure formed over the area of the "tail-bone" which are prone to infection.

PINWORMS: The most common parasitic worm found in humans in the United States.

PLAGUE: Pandemic infectious disease caused by the bacteria Yersinia pestis.

PLASMID: A repository of genetic material used by bacteria for special functions, such as antibiotic resistance.

PLEOMORPHS: Bacteria with variable shapes.

PNEUMONIA: An infection of the lower respiratory tract.

PNEUMONIC PLAGUE: An extremely virulent form of Plague that affects the lungs.

PRIMARY INTENTION: Wound healing aided by closure with sutures, staples, glues, or other method.

PROGNOSIS: A forecast of the probable outcome of a disease.

PROKARYOTE: a microscopic single-celled organism that has neither a distinct nucleus with a membrane nor other specialized organelles. Prokaryotes include the bacteria and cyanobacteria.

PROTISTS: A group of organisms consisting of protozoa, unicellular algae, and slime molds.

PROTOZOA: Organisms, usually single-celled eukaryotes, living in water or as parasites.

PROTOZOAN: Singular form of "protozoa."

PYELONEPHRITIS: Infection of the kidneys.

REGIMEN: A prescribed way to take a medicine for a certain infection or condition.

RESERVOIR: Any person, animal, plant, soil or substance in which an infectious agent normally lives and multiplies.

RESISTANCE: The ability of a microbe to counteract the effect of an antibiotic.

RIBOSOME: An organelle in bacteria that functions to synthesize proteins.

RICKETS: A deformity of long bones in young children due to Vitamin D deficiency; not an infectious disease.

RICKETTSIA: A subgroup of bacterial species that must enter a host cell to reproduce.

ROCKY MOUNTAIN SPOTTED FEVER: infectious disease spread by the bites of ticks.

SCARLET FEVER: Infectious disease caused by group A Strep characterized by fever and a bright red rash.

SEBACEOUS CYST: A swelling of a skin gland associated with hair follicles.

SEBUM: Oily material associated with skin glands.

SECONDARY INTENTION: The natural healing process of an open wound over time.

SEDATIVE: A drug taken for its calming or sleep-inducing effect.

SEPSIS: a generalized toxic state resulting from the spread of bacteria or their toxins from a focus of infection

SEPTICEMIA: An infection of the blood.

SEPTICEMIC PLAGUE: A form of plague that invades the circulation.

SHELF LIFE EXTENSION PROGRAM: A program of the U.S. Department of Defense and FDA to evaluate the potency of drugs after their expiration dates.

SHIGA: A toxin produced by a virulent strain of E. coli known as 0157:H7.

SHORT-TERM IMMUNITY: The body's immediate response to a threat; also, the transfer of antibodies via injection of serum or through breastfeeding.

SIDE EFFECT: A secondary effect of a drug, usually an adverse reaction.

SINUSITIS: Inflammation of the spaces in the bones of the face and skull.

SOCIAL DISTANCING: The strategy of avoiding close contact with others in epidemic outbreaks.

SPECULUM: An instrument used to visualize an orifice or canal in the body such as the vagina or nasal cavity.

SPIRILLI: Curved or spiral-shaped bacteria.

SPIROCHETE: A term for a spiral-shaped bacterium such as the one seen in syphilis infections.

SPORES: A dormant or reproductive body produced by some microorganisms and capable of development into a new individual.

SPUTUM: Material coughed up from the respiratory tract.

STERILE SALINE: Mixture of water and salt which, once boiled, is used as a solution to clean open wounds.

STREP THROAT: A common bacterial infection of the throat caused by Streptococcus pyogenes (group A Strep).

STREPTOCOCCUS PNEUMONIAE: The most common type of bacterial pneumonia; sometimes called "pneumococcal pneumonia."

STYE: An infection of blocked glands near the eyelash.

SUBCLINICAL INFECTION: An infection that is nearly or completely without physical signs or symptoms; seen in "carriers" of diseases that transmit illness but aren't sick themselves.

SUSPENSION: The mixing of an antibiotic with a liquid for pediatric use; an elixir.

SYPHILIS: A sexually transmitted disease caused by the spirochete Treponema pallidum.

SYSTEMIC INFECTION: an infection in which the pathogen invades the entire body rather than just one area or organ.

TACHYCARDIA: An elevated heart rate (above 100).

TETANUS: Infection caused by the bacterium Clostridium tetani.

TINEA CORPORIS: Fungal infection commonly known as "ringworm."

TINEA PEDIS: Fungal infection commonly known as "athlete's foot."

TOXIN: a harmful substance produced by a living organism.

TRAVELER'S DIARRHEA: Inflammation of the small intestine often caused by a virulent strain of E. coli.

TROPHOZOITE: The active form of the parasite *Giardia lamblia* and other protozoans.

TUBERCULOSIS: A contagious disease caused by Mycobacterium tuberculosis, usually affecting the lungs.

TYPHOID FEVER: Epidemic infection caused by the bacteria Salmonella typhi in contaminated and undercooked food.

TYPHUS: A Rickettsial infection characterized by rashes and high fevers.

UMBILICUS: The navel or "belly button."

URGENCY: A sensation of having to urinate.

VECTOR: An organism that transmits a disease or parasite from one animal or plant to another.

VERTIGO: a sensation of spinning and loss of balance caused by disease affecting the inner ear.

VETERINARY EQUIVALENT: A medicine used in animals that is identical in ingredients, dosage, and appearance to the same medicine used in humans.

VIRION: The infectious form of a virus as it exists outside the host cell.

VIRULENT: Harmful in its effects; capable of causing disease.

VIRUSES: Infective agents that are able to multiply only within the living cells of a host.

WHIPWORM: A parasitic worm that uses a human as a host.

WHOOPING COUGH: Highly contagious disease characterized by coughing fits followed by a high-pitched "whoop" sound during inhalation.

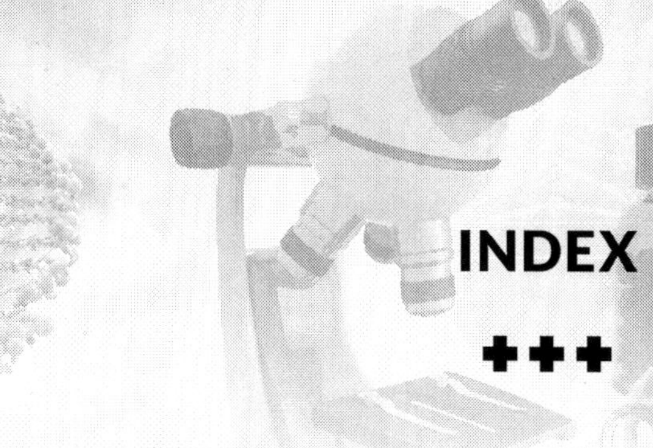

INDEX

✚✚✚

C

F

G

H

I

J

K

L

M

N

O

T

U

V

W

Y

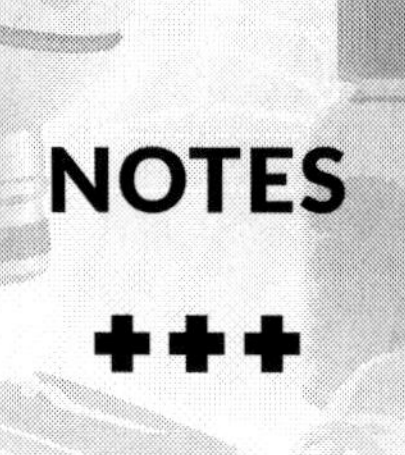

NOTES

✚✚✚

NOTES

NOTES

Made in the USA
Coppell, TX
20 August 2023